T0073126

Treating Eczema with Traditional Chinese Medicine

Treating Eczema with Traditional Chinese Medicine

Xiu-Min Li
New York Medical College, USA

Henry Ehrlich
asthmaallergieschildren.com

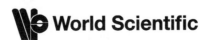

World Scientific

NEW JERSEY · LONDON · SINGAPORE · BEIJING · SHANGHAI · HONG KONG · TAIPEI · CHENNAI · TOKYO

Published by

World Scientific Publishing Co. Pte. Ltd.

5 Toh Tuck Link, Singapore 596224

USA office: 27 Warren Street, Suite 401-402, Hackensack, NJ 07601

UK office: 57 Shelton Street, Covent Garden, London WC2H 9HE

Library of Congress Cataloging-in-Publication Data

Names: Li, Xiu-Min, author. | Ehrlich, Henry, 1949– author.
Title: Treating eczema with traditional Chinese medicine / Xiu-Min Li,
    New York Medical College, USA, Henry Ehrlich, asthmaallergieschildren.com.
Description: First edition. | New Jersey : World Scientific, [2022] |
    Includes bibliographical references and index.
Identifiers: LCCN 2021043871 | ISBN 9789811245923 (hardcover) |
    ISBN 9789811247538 (paperback) | ISBN 9789811245930 (ebook) |
    ISBN 9789811245947 (ebook other)
Subjects: LCSH: Eczema--Alternative treatment. | Medicine, Chinese.
Classification: LCC RL251 .L5 2022 | DDC 616.5/1--dc23/eng/20211028
LC record available at https://lccn.loc.gov/2021043871

British Library Cataloguing-in-Publication Data
A catalogue record for this book is available from the British Library.

For any available supplementary material, please visit
https://www.worldscientific.com/worldscibooks/10.1142/12519#t=suppl

ABOUT THE AUTHOR

Dr. Xiu-Min Li

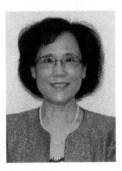 Dr. Xiu-Min Li is a full professor in the Departments of Pathology, Immunology and Microbiology, and Otolaryngology at New York Medical College/ Westchester Medical Center. She has pioneered research into the efficacy, safety and mechanisms of traditional Chinese medicine (TCM), for immune disorders. Her research has been funded by the NIH, industry, private foundations, and family donations with over 100 publications in these fields. Dr. Li obtained her medical degree at the Henan University of Chinese Medicine (Zhengzhou and a Master's degree in Clinical Pediatric Immunology from the Graduate School of the China Academy of Chinese Medical Sciences (Beijing). She worked as an Attending Pediatrician at China-Japan Friendship Hospital (Beijing). She was a Visiting Scientist at Stanford and postdoctoral fellow in Clinical Immunology at Johns Hopkins where she was appointed Instructor in 1997. Dr. Li joined the Division of Pediatric Allergy and Immunology at Mount Sinai when it was established in 1997, where she rose to the rank of tenured Professor. She has chaired prominent committees about the use of alternative medicines for allergic diseases at the American Academy of Allergy, Asthma & Immunology (AAAAI) and internationally and is the recipient of the Future of Health Technology Award in Cambridge, Mass. in 2016 and the Novel Research in Chinese Medicine Overseas Award in Beijing in 2017.

CONTENTS

FOREWORD

Anne Maitland, MD, PhD*

Can the practitioner's art be grafted on the main trunk of the fundamental sciences in such a way that there shall arise a symmetrical growth, like an expanding tree, the leaves of which may be for the "healing of the nations"?

Francis Peabody[1]

As a physician, researcher, teacher, and mentor, Dr. Francis Peabody was a bona fide superhero of the golden age of medicine. After his chief residency at Peter Bent Brigham Hospital in Boston, attending physician efforts at Johns Hopkins and Rockefeller Hospital, experience as a World War I Army field doctor, and as one of the founding editors of the *Journal of Clinical Investigation*, Dr. Peabody also helped set up the first modern medical school in China. He spoke of impressing "the value of Western medicine ... on a population who prefer to rely on the native system of practice ...". That is, Dr. Peabody and his colleagues, in the newly established Department of Medicine at the Peking Union Medical College, hoped to instill the scientific method of Western medicine into a culture that utilized the ancient arts of Traditional Chinese Medicine (TCM): acupuncture, herbal products and movement exercises.

This was a tense courtship. In a 1922 *Science* article, Peabody observed that the Chinese "like Western surgery but they do not care for Western

*Dr. Anne Maitland received her MD and PhD from the University of Pennsylvania and did her allergy and immunology fellowship at Brigham and Women's Hospital and Mount Sinai Hospital in New York, NY. She practices in Tarrytown, NY.

medicine."[2] With "new ways to peer into the body, new medications and pathogen-free surgeries", "the practitioners of Western medicine — for the most part missionaries — [provided ready relief] to an enormous burden of traumatic injuries, infections and large superficial tumors". Western "medicine" failed to win over the Chinese people. To understand reticence on the part of Chinese patients, Dr. Peabody had to look no further than the emerging attitudes of his fellow "scientific" Western clinicians, towards many of their patients, and not only in China. "He witnessed too many colleagues, both community and academic clinicians, 'giving up' on their patients, if vague symptoms of pain and fatigue did not fall into diagnostic box or respond to the latest modern therapies. Peabody estimated that he and his colleagues held clinics in which approximately half of their patients complained of symptoms for which an adequate organic cause could not be discovered."[1]

> A wise man should consider that health is the Greatest of human blessings and learn how by his own thought to derive benefit from his illness.
>
> Hippocrates

A few years after his amazing accomplishments in the US and China, Dr. Peabody became incurably ill, and "suddenly, this legendary physician was a patient himself". These lessons, on the other side of the bench and bedside, presented an opportunity that this die-hard teacher couldn't pass up sharing with his students and the Harvard Medical School. In his classic essay, "The care of the patient", Dr. Peabody urges the following: (1) the importance of individualizing medical care, lifting the patient above the sea of statistics and mounting literature; (2) be aware of "the dehumanizing experience of patients" while treating ailments and "to not forget [to treat] the person and not the disease"; and (3), for "patients who have symptoms for which an organic cause cannot be determined, … [and] likely constitute up to half of any physician's practice", tend to the patient's emotional needs, as the patient copes with chronic illness and the pursuit to understand the etiology of the illness is unmasked.

> It is rather fashionable to say that the modern physician has become "too scientific" [or] not scientific enough? The popular conception of a scientist

as a man who works in a laboratory and who uses instruments of precision is as inaccurate as it is superficial, for a scientist is known, not by his technical processes, but by his intellectual processes; and the essence of the scientific method of thought is that it proceeds in an orderly manner toward the establishment of a truth.

Francis Peabody[1]

Before becoming incurably ill and delivering his series of lectures on the goals and efforts of the caring physician scientist,[3] Dr. Peabody helped plant the seeds of Western scientific medicine in the rich Chinese soil of Traditional Herbal Medicine, to not only fight disease, but also prevent it. As an attending physician in Peking Union Medical College, Francis Peabody introduced the scientific method to Chinese physicians and nurses. He knew that Western-trained Chinese nationals, whether they received their training at home or abroad, had to be the ambassadors, "grafting" the fundamentals of the scientific method onto the time-tested, cornerstone of the ancient Eastern healing arts — TCM.

Nearly a century later, Dr. Xiu-Min Li, who was trained in both traditions in China before embarking on a research career in the United States, embodies much of what I believe Dr. Peabody envisioned. A caring physician, diligent and visionary scientist, provocative teacher and mentor to many, including her former trainee (yours truly), Dr. Li has been unlocking the secrets of TCM, with rigorous scientific pursuits, to address the first pandemic of the 21st century — allergen-triggered mast cell activation disorders (commonly referred to "allergies"), from a nuisance of a condition, rhinitis — the number two reason children miss school and adults call in sick — to difficult-to-treat eczema and the rising tide of food allergies, asthma and anaphylaxis.[4] Prior to the COVID-19 pandemic, studies revealed that nearly 1 of 50 Americans have been treated for anaphylaxis to food and medications, for example, and many more carry epinephrine auto-injectors, while social distancing to avoid triggers of these hypersensitivity disorders.

At the bench at New York Medical College in collaboration with colleagues in China and other nations, Dr. Li and her team are decoding the components of TCM herbs with anti-inflammatory properties as potent at corticosteroids as well as other pharmaceutical grade anti-inflammatory agents. Modern-day living has exposed many of us to chemicals and physical elements that disrupt the connectivity of our borders — the skin and the linings of the respiratory, gastro-intestinal and urogenital tract and associated immune and neuronal components — leaving patients isolated and desperate for relief. At the bedside and in the lab, Dr. Li is restoring the balance of the triad of these three organ systems, one patient at a time. And, in this volume, one will learn the latest of Dr. Li's efforts to elevate the ancient healing ways of TCM and acupuncture, to treat and prevent hypersensitivity disorders, where the efficacy of traditional Western therapeutics have plateaued, concentrating on that most common and stubborn of conditions — eczema. Combining her experience of TCM and the scientific method of Western medicine, the clinical practice of Dr. Xiu-Min Li is "science", as Stephen Paget stated in 1909, "touched with emotion".[5]

References

1. Peabody FW. The care of the patient. *JAMA*. 1927;88(12):877–882. doi:10.1001/jama.1927.02680380001001
2. Peabody FW. The Department of Medicine at the Peking Union Medical College. *Science*. 1922;56(1447):317–320. Retrieved from https://www.jstor.org/stable/1647620
3. Lavizzo-Mourey R. The secret of patient care. *National Scientific Meeting, Society of General Internal Medicine*. 2006. Retrieved from http://www.ramcampaign.org/pages/documents/riza_bylined_article.pdf
4. Platts-Mills TA. The allergy epidemics: 1870–2010. *J Allergy Clin Immunol*. 2015;136: 3–13.
5. Lenfant C. Clinical research to clinical practice — Lost in translation? *N Engl J Med*. 2003;349:868–874.

Suggested Further Reading

Peking Union Medical College. *Science*. 1922;56(1450):410–411. Retrieved from https://www.jstor.org/stable/1648105

Rabin PL, Rabin D. The care of the patient: Francis Peabody revisited. *JAMA*. 1984;252(6):819–820. doi: 10.1001/jama.1984.03350060063033.

Ross MA. Physicians and patients, then and now. *BC Medical Journal*. 2007;49(8):429–435. Retrieved from https://bcmj.org/premise/physicians-and-patients-then-and-now

Part I
Research

"GIVE-UP PATIENTS": THE ROAD TO ECZEMA TREATMENT

A CONVERSATION WITH DR. XIU-MIN LI

Henry Ehrlich*

1) Why did you choose to specialize in eczema care when you founded your practice?

Severe eczema was an important unmet need in American medicine. I approached my former chairman at the Mount Sinai School of Medicine and my mentor Dr. Hugh Sampson at the Jaffe Food Allergy Institute about opening an off-site clinic to treat it. Dr. Sampson, who is a powerful figure in the field of allergies, particularly food allergies, had expressed frustration over eczema in his practice. He and I visited China-Japan Friendship Hospital, where my former mentor spoke favorably about my treatment of children with eczema, G.I. disorders, and recurrent respiratory infections, which are very common in China because of the climate and the environment.

---

*Henry Ehrlich is author of two other books about the work of Dr. Li—*Food Allergies: Tradtional Chinese Medicine, Western Science, and the Search for a Cure*, and (with Dr. Li) *Traditional Chinese Medicine, Western Science, and the Fight Against Allergic Disease*.

After the clinic opened, Dr. Sampson sent me two patients whom he called "give-up" patients. Discouraged with the topical-steroid cycle that characterizes eczema treatment, Dr. Sampson had raised the possibility of alternative medicine to these patients, and they leapt at it.

It was August 1, a time when New York children are generally wearing shorts and short-sleeved shirts. My first patient was 18 months old and dressed more appropriately for late fall. When we took off his clothes, I saw why. He was covered head-to-toe with oozing, staph-infected lesions, which he promptly began to scratch. That explained the overdressing — it was the only deterrent to scratching.

I had expected quick resolution using oral medication — teas — based on my experience in China. I wasn't prepared for this level of severity. In addition to the eczema, which was being treated with steroids, he also had allergies to 20 or 30 foods.

The first thing I did was to give him acupressure, which involves compressing the skin at key points on the body. This quieted him down and he stopped scratching. I said to the mother that this would soon wear off. Acupuncture would last longer, but small children are not usually receptive to it. Nevertheless, she asked me to try, and the child was quite cooperative.

I sent them off with the teas and we set another appointment for four weeks. During the interval I went to the TCM literature, both classical and contemporary. I had a good idea what I was looking for and by the time they returned, I was ready for them with a protocol of creams and bath in addition to the oral medication. Within weeks the child's skin was well on the way to being normal and within a year, he began to tolerate some of the food allergens.

2)   Was this little boy typical of your early patients?

Yes. Their doctors had exhausted the treatments they were familiar with, and the patients had given up on themselves. The children would cry and so would their mothers. The whole family would be suffering from sleeplessness. Teenagers felt that they had lost their lives. With adult patients it was the same thing. After just a few weeks of treatment, they would start crying again: "Why didn't I find you a year earlier?"

3) Were your colleagues receptive to this new method?

Like Dr. Sampson, many of them were frustrated at their inability to treat these patients. A fellow made a presentation on the case to a luncheon of pediatricians at Mount Sinai, and one by one I began receiving referrals from the doctors who had attended, mostly for children who were steroid dependent. From there my team prepared an abstract for presentation at the American Academy of Allergy, Asthma, and Immunology (AAAAI) and we were on the map.

4) What accounts for your concentration on eczema?

The main reason was that it interested me. Another reason was that I knew from my experience in Beijing when I worked in China-Japan Friendship Hospital that we could get good responses to treatment. We didn't use steroids. Some tea and a little cream. Yet, I knew that my colleagues in America struggled with it. I had been under the impression that it was quite easy to treat and I could have an impact. I wasn't prepared for what I saw.

It wasn't just the extent of the disease. It was also the toll it took on family quality of life. Kids were crying. Mothers were crying. They were all sleeping badly. Most of these families also had bad food allergies, but food allergy is a silent disease. People worry about it, but with eczema they suffer every day. You see it. It can be quantified using two systems. One is called the SCORing Atopic Dermatitis (SCORAD) index that "combines body surface area measurements with signs of intensity, and symptoms of itch and sleeplessness, to calculate a score of 0–103 for disease severity". [1]

The sites affected by eczema are shaded on a drawing of a body. The rule of 9 is used to calculate the affected area (A) as a percentage of the whole body.

- Head and neck 9%
- Upper limbs 9% each
- Lower limbs 18% each
- Anterior trunk 18%
- Back 18%
- 1% for genitals

The score for each area is added up. The total area is "A", which has a possible maximum of 100%.

A representative area of eczema is selected. In this area, the intensity of each of the following signs is assessed as none (0), mild (1), moderate (2), or severe (3).

- Redness
- Swelling
- Oozing/crusting
- Scratch marks
- Skin thickening (lichenification)
- Dryness (this is assessed in an area where there is no inflammation)

The other is called the Dermatology Quality of Life (DQOL) index: ten questions that help assess the impact of the disease on a scale from 0 to 30. The questions not only encompass physical symptoms, such as pain and itching, but also behavior, choice of wardrobe, and social and sexual activity.

In an early retrospective study of 14 patients, during the first three months of treatment, 7 patients experienced from 60–90% improvement (classified as "good") and sustained it over 3 to 15 months of follow-up. One patient achieved excellent improvement (>90%) in the first 3 months, which was sustained for 5.4 months, the last report before the study was written up. Seven patients showed inadequate (<60%) improvement in SCORAD in the first 1–3 months but attained good or excellent improvement over the following 3 to 15 months. At the end of the study period, 12 patients had sustained good (>60%) improvement, and 5 out of 14 had sustained excellent improvement (>90%). Improved quality of life, especially improvements in sleep and pruritus, were observed sooner than improvements in skin quality and SCORAD. Eleven of 14 patients experienced at least a 50% improvement in quality of life during the first 1–3 months of therapy. At the end of the study period, 12 of 14 patients reported sustained improvement in quality of life with 10 of 14 reporting >80% improvement.[2]

The real reward can't be quantified. Happiness and relief can't be measured. And they were very real.

5) Did you have a treatment framework in mind to begin with or did you search through the TCM literature for ideas?

The framework was there. While the severity of disease I encountered was far worse than what I had seen in China, when I worked in China-Japan Friendship Hospital I still had ideas about where to go based on knowledge and experience. I studied both TCM and Western medicine in China. Since coming to the US, I had also trained in food allergy and immunology. This was the framework. I had been collecting TCM books since medical school. Every time I went to China, I would come back with as many texts as I could carry and shipped even more. I also began to build my lab, which allowed us to study the underlying mechanisms of eczema and the therapies, along with our work on food allergies and asthma, for which I have also developed treatments.

6) Has anything about the eczema epidemic surprised you?

The nature of the disease has changed. Topical steroid addiction and withdrawal are diseases caused by medical treatment. As I said, we didn't see them in China. The short-term relief from the discomfort of eczema afforded by the topical steroids is irresistible. It's too easy when that itch starts or that lesion reappears to just rub on some more cream.

It's also too easy to overlook the other organ systems that are involved in eczema. Patient ages have gotten lower and lower. Five years ago, I mostly saw teenagers and adults who suffer the unsightly and painful condition known as red-skin syndrome. Now more and more of them are very young children whose parents relied on steroids to temporarily relieve their children's suffering by overusing the creams. I don't blame them. Patient suffering disrupts the whole household. Another disturbing problem is that steroids are sometimes hidden in cosmetics. I have had several patients like this.

The worst cases are receiving immune suppressants like cyclosporine, which are used to keep transplant patients from rejecting their new organs. Their skin is badly damaged and painful.

7)   What is the history of your treatment? I know that some of it was based on Tang Dynasty (618–907 CE) treatments for burns and wounds. How much did that early history figure in your thinking?

It's true that some of it comes from that era, which was when gunpowder was invented. That is only for the surface damage, similar to first or second-degree burns, and stopping infection. But eczema is a multi-organ, multi-system disease. The Song Dynasty (960–1279 CE) was more important. The pediatrician Qian Yi wrote a book called *Famous Formulations for Pediatric Disease*, which is still popular. These books emphasized not just the appearance of the skin but patient emotions. We have to remember digestion and mood.

Today I read these books through the lens of modern chemistry and pharmacology. I studied about 200 formulations and the herbs they contained and had to check the FDA website to see which ones had warnings. It's important to know that some herbs that carry warnings in the U.S. are used every day in TCM in China without any problem. The most famous example is *Ma Huang*, which has been used to safely control asthma for thousands of years. In this country it is a considered a precursor to methamphetamine. But anything can be a poison in large enough quantities. Licorice is a powerful therapeutic as well as a flavoring, but it can be poisonous in excessive quantities.

8)   How did you arrive at your triple therapy?

Everything I did was driven by knowledge, experience and lots of reading from old and new texts. There were several goals. To relieve itching. To heal skin. To restore digestive health. To rebalance the immune system. Some inflammation is a good thing. It helps us fight infection. But with bad eczema, inflammation goes too far. Uncontrollable scratching damages the skin where staph infection can establish itself. Just reducing inflammation is not enough. Topical steroids accomplish that, but the relief is only temporary. The inflammation rebounds, leading to topical steroid addiction. Remedying all this couldn't be accomplished with a single medicine that can be taken by mouth or injected. From the thousands of years of TCM, I developed a regimen of baths to hydrate the skin as well as medicate, creams to protect and soothe the skin as well as medicate, and oral teas. They combine anti-bacterial, anti-fungal, and anti-inflammatory properties. They are absorbed into the system through a variety of pathways because just one is not enough to achieve a therapeutic effect. They can be used by infants as well as older patients. All my medications have a high safety profile.

9) How important is it to stick strictly to the protocols? I know from interviewing many of your eczema patients that when they start to feel "normal", they slip, and have a setback. How do you deal with them?

Eczema, food intolerance/food allergy, and environmental allergies are different conditions, but can co-exist and make truly healing the skin very difficult. Severe eczema is a physical disease but it's also a lifestyle disease affecting the whole family as well as the individual. Even after the skin is outwardly clear, patients remain vulnerable not only to food and environmental allergens but also to behavioral triggers, such as excessive physical activity. At this stage, the individuals and families should continue their established protocol on food and environmental exposure until what I call Phase I (See Chapter 12) is achieved. It will give the individual a time to build immunological tolerance before the most significant changes in resetting the immune system are achieved by following the milestone plan. It sounds simple but is not easy to process and requires strong determination by individual patients and their entire support systems. Exposing the patient to previously avoided foods, environmental allergens, and exercise or work too soon may overwhelm the immune system. Once this happens, getting back to "normal" again will take longer. The two rules for full-speed skin healing are: 1) Stay on the protocol; 2) Continue lifestyle discipline; don't overdo it no matter how good you may feel.

10) Do you have any thoughts about the allergic march, also known as the atopic march, which generally recognizes eczema as the first allergic disease, followed by some combination of food allergies, asthma and allergic rhinitis? Since eczematous skin is considered the first induction point for some allergens, we wonder whether that progression might be stopped by treating the skin. What is your feeling about TCM's potential for halting it? Can TCM help stave off development of more allergies?

This is only possible in the first four months of life, when "naïve" patients' exposure to the environment is very limited, mostly to what they touch and what they consume in breast milk or formula. If the skin barrier is strong, it is largely impermeable to outside antigens. But if it is weak, antigens such as peanut residue and dust mites can present to the immune system, starting the process of sensitization that can lead to development of true allergies.

Unfortunately, the literature is limited on this. It's hard to study prevention because by the time you know someone is prone to allergy, they already are showing symptoms. Research money is very short for prophylaxis and weighted towards treatment. This makes sense because how do you find a study population before they are symptomatic? By then, they are likely to be on steroids, which upset the immune system even further than it already is after chronic use. The sensitivity spreads from one epithelial organ to another, from skin to digestion to airways.

I am in a unique position to treat and study this population because I have many very young patients and they have younger siblings. The parents bring these infants to me to try to stop further disease progression. We use blood tests to study biomarkers as we do to all other patients. And we treat them with creams and baths. No teas at a young age. These botanical medications are easy to administer to very young children, and their effect is quick. They effectively restore the barrier function of the skin and the natural balance of Th1 and Th2 acquired immunity before chronic disease is well established.

11)   Your vision for years has been to provide treatment within the context of "integrative medicine". Could you explain what that means at this point in your career and how much progress you are making?

All patients receive primary and specialty care from allopathic physicians who order their tests for my practice. Most of these doctors are comfortable working with me and many of them have referred patients. That was not the case when I began, but most doctors care about their patients and when they can't give them relief, they are open to alternatives, as is the case with eczema and overuse of topical steroids, some asthma cases, and food allergies. There are also allergists who specialize in treating food allergies with oral immunotherapy (OIT) and sublingual immunotherapy (SLIT). While I also treat food allergy, I think that OIT and SLIT can accelerate the process. However, these methods can cause symptoms, 90 percent of which are gastric. I can treat these reactions. I call it "calming the immune system". Some prominent OIT and SLIT specialists recommend our practice to patients and I refer our patients to them.

Eventually, I would like to help these partner-doctors treat the various components of allergic diseases as part of a whole system. Controlling eczema with steroids in support of OIT doesn't address immune stress that is simmering underneath.

But I would like other doctors to be able to treat certain patients without regularly consulting me. This book is a step towards that, I hope. Our eczema protocol is very safe and straightforward.

Ultimately, we need to train more practitioners to do the TCM component without my being routinely involved, which I hope to do through a foundation that has been on paper for years, but there's only so much time and money. The pandemic didn't help.

One very exciting new development is that I have been asked to become a consulting physician to a group of otolaryngologists (ENTS). These doctors are frequently called on to treat conditions that have significant co-morbidities that are allergic in nature, including eczema, asthma and food allergies. My friend and colleague Dr. Paul Ehrlich will provide mainstream allergy support preparatory to my seeing them. He has been referring patients to me for many years whose condition he judges to be beyond the scope of conventional allergy practice. Together with the ENTs, I hope to forge a practice network that will benefit more patients and spread knowledge of this approach to integrative medicine.

References

1.   SCORAD — Codes and concepts. Available at http://www.dermnetnz.org/dermatitis/scorad.html
2.   Thanik E, Wisniewski JA, Nowak-Wegrzyn A, Sampson H, Li XM. Improvement of skin lesions and life quality in moderate-to-severe eczema patients by combined TCM therapy. *Ann Allergy Asthma Immunol.* 2018;121(1):135e136.

2

THE ALLERGIST'S DILEMMA

Paul Ehrlich, MD*

Of the allergic diseases I have treated for 40-plus years, the one that has given me the most anguish is eczema. Uncontrolled asthma is the most lethal, but it can largely be treated. Allergic rhinitis is the most annoying to patients, but antihistamines blunt symptoms and we have cured many patients with injections. Food allergies cause the most worry, but they are generally asymptomatic and can be contained by avoidance and emergency medication. Eczema, however, while not life-threatening, causes the most routine misery. It is painful to patients, and their misery is on display for the world's prying eyes. The sight of a teenage girl sobbing in my consulting room and talking about suicide is heartbreaking.

I always measure progress in allergy treatment by a standard set by my old colleague at Walter Reed Medical Center, Dr. Arnold Levinson, who spent most of his subsequent career at the University of Pennsylvania. Ten

---

*Dr. Paul Ehrlich trained in pediatrics at Bellevue Hospital at NYU, and did his allergy and immunology fellowship at Walter Reed Army Medical Center. He is a long-practicing allergist in New York City, Past-President of the New York Allergy and Asthma Society, and co-author of *Asthma Allergies Children: A Parent's Guide.*

years ago, he asked an audience of 300 allergists if they could name a true advance in asthma treatment since the development of inhaled corticosteroids in the 1940s. No one raised a hand. He could also have asked about the emergence of topical steroids to treat eczema in the 1950s.

We are fortunate that in the past decade a few breakthroughs have been made, some topical and some injectable, both for eczema and asthma. Whether they will reach the status of go-to medications the way steroids have remains to be seen. I can say that in the short term the intricacies of prescribing them and paying for them will impede their universal administration and, if the example of topical steroids teaches us anything, to their overuse.

Two cases stand out for me after all this time. One was a ten-year old girl who arrived in my office after years of bouncing from one teaching hospital to another presenting with lesions "everywhere", her face, neck, eyelids, and down to her feet. She was so self-conscious that she didn't want to go to school. She couldn't sleep through the night. Her friends thought she had polka-dot sheets because they were bloody from her scratching.[1]

Another was a six-year-old boy whose skin was so dire that his parents were afraid to fly with him for fear of alarming other passengers. He couldn't walk. I had to carry him to my consulting room.

Both these cases had happy endings, and the common thread was the ability to partner in treatment with Dr. Xiu-Min Li. I sent the girl to her. I knew the limits of what conventional allergy could accomplish. Xiu-Min sent the little boy to me because she wanted to know if I, along with a distinguished dermatologist who practiced down the hall, thought there was any more to be done from the allopathic side. Over the years we have shared many patients. I do what I can, based on my training and experience. She does what she does, and it sometimes seems like a miracle. If I only had another 20 years... Fortunately, I have met many eager medical students who share that ambition. My hope is that they will carry this medical legacy forward.

Reference

1.   Ehrlich H. *Food Allergies: Traditional Chinese Medicine, Western Science, and the Search for a Cure.* Third Avenue Books, 2014.

TRADITIONAL CHINESE MEDICINE FOR FOOD ALLERGY AND ECZEMA[b]

Zixi Wang, MD[*,†,a], Zhen-Zhen Wang, PhD[‡,§,a],
Jan Geliebter, PhD[§,¶], Raj Tiwari, PhD[§,¶], and
Xiu-Min Li, MD, MS[§]

[*] *Department of Allergy, Peking Union Medical College Hospital,*
Beijing 100730, China
[†] *Beijing Key Laboratory of Precision Medicine for Diagnosis and*
Treatment of Allergic Diseases, Beijing 100730, China
[‡] *College of Academy of Chinese Medicine Sciences,*
Henan University of Chinese Medicine, Zhengzhou 450056, China
[§] *Department of Pathology, Microbiology and Immunology,*
and Department of Otolaryngology
New York Medical College, Valhalla, New York 10595, USA

---

[a] These authors contributed equally to this manuscript.
[b] This article was published in the *Ann Allergy Clin Immunol.* 2021 Jun;126(6):639–654 and is reprinted with permission.

Correspondence to: Xiu-Min Li, New York Medical College, Valhalla, New York 10595, USA. Email: XiuMin_Li@nymc.edu

Keywords: Food allergy, traditional Chinese medicine, food allergy herbal formula-2 (FAHF-2), EB-FAHF-2, eczema, atopic dermatitis.

Introduction

FA Burden, Unmet Need, and CAM Use

Food allergy (FA) has increased over several decades affecting approximately 10% of both American children[1] and adults.[2] Overall economic costs of food allergy were estimated at $24.8 billion annually in United States ($4184 per year per child).[3] FA is an immune-mediated, potentially life-threatening adverse reaction comprising IgE-mediated immediate hypersensitivity reactions, delayed non-IgE-mediated reactions, and disorders combining both IgE-mediated and non-IgE-mediated immune pathways. Th2 cytokines are central in pathogenesis of IgE mediated FA reactions. IgE memory response due to long-lived IgE$^+$ plasma cells contributes to persistent food antigen-specific IgE production, and FA chronicity.[4] Non IgE-mediated FA includes gastrointestinal disorders such as food protein-induced enterocolitis syndrome [FPIES][5] — an overreactive TNF-α, IL-8 and tryptase response, and a deficit in TGF-β1.[5] Currently, there is only one FDA-approved treatment — Palforzia, a well-defined peanut allergen powder — that increases immune tolerance to peanut. This is a milestone, although reactions are a challenge. Strict allergen avoidance and rescue medication — the major treatment strategies — present organizational and social challenges.[6] Therefore, methods to prevent and cure severe reactions are needed. Complementary and alternative medicine (CAM) is one potential approach. CAM for FA rose from 2002 (11%) to 2006 (18%).[7] In 2016, the American Academy of Allergy, Asthma, and Immunology reported that FA has been one of the most common indications for CAM use (53.6%).[8] Traditional Chinese medicine (TCM) is a major CAM modality in the United States. TCM is viewed as system medicine, sharing a concept with Japanese and Korean traditional medicine. TCM is one of the world's oldest medical practices. Asian countries have used it for thousands of years for various health conditions including gastrointestinal and skin systems. Although there was no term for FA in the ancient Chinese medicine, Wu Mei Wan was formulated by an ancient TCM physician (Zhang, Zhongjing) to fight intestinal parasites, which we now know elicit an IgE response, suggesting use for alleviating similar reactions to foods. Although the Western image of Chinese medicine comes from storefronts with jars of herbs, TCM and integrative medicine are part of mainstream Asian medical education. They are practiced in the major hospitals in mainland China, Taiwan, Japan, and Korea, where modern laboratory science and data-mining capabilities such as systems pharmacology and in silico docking are unlocking ancient formulations to treat contemporary maladies. With this kind of scientific validation, coupled with patient demand for natural alternatives, this approach is likely to play a larger role in the West. Costs are normally covered by insurance in Asia, the European Union, and the UK.[9] Extensive clinical trials are yet to be performed, but preclinical studies of TCM herbal formulas suggest an exciting potential for FA.[9]

Eczema Burden, Unmet Need, and Use of TCM

Eczema is a common allergic inflammatory skin disorder characterized by itchy, scaly, erythematous, and oozing skin, affecting up to 20% of children and 1–3% of adults in most countries.[10] Estimates of US costs range from $364 million to $3.8 billion per year.[11] Allergic rhinitis, FA, and asthma are frequently co-morbid with eczema. Increased risks of infection, lymphoma, pruritus, and nonmelanoma skin cancer have also been reported in atopic dermatitis (AD) patients.[12] Eczema pathogenesis is associated with multiple genetic and environmental factors. Immune cells such as eosinophils, mast cells, and cytokines such as Th2 (IL-4, IL-5, IL-13 and IL-31), Th17 (IL-17A, IL-17F, IL-22 and IL-26), and Th9 cells play important roles in different stages of the disease.[13] Topical corticosteroids (steroids) are first-line treatment; however, over time, AD becomes steroid refractory in some patients. About 10% of them require one or more systemic treatments.[14]

Sudden steroid withdrawal results in sleep disturbance, extreme itching, painful skin, and stress, which are mediated by complex inflammatory cell and cytokine networks and altered skin integrity. FDA-approved non-steroid treatments include dupilumab injection (biologic), topical crisaborole ointment (phosphodiesterase 4 inhibitor) and topical tacrolimus ointment, and pimecrolimus cream (calcineurin inhibitors). Dupilumab, an IL-4/IL-13 receptor blockade, is costly, and psoriasis has been observed as a rare side effect.[15] Crisaborole is only recommended for mild-to-moderate disorders.[16] Thus, AD currently represents an important unmet health care need. TCM was used to treat skin diseases for centuries before the introduction of Western medicine. Published TCM studies over the past 20 years have shown efficacy in treating eczema patients, including young children, with no serious adverse effects, improving severity scores, reducing pruritus, achieving better quality of life, and decreasing corticosteroid use.[17] In this paper, we review the past ten years of AD-TCM clinical studies and investigations for the underlying mechanisms. Although food allergy and eczema are different, comorbidity in children is common.[18] Chronic eczema may create vulnerability in children to conditions including food allergy (allergy march). Food allergy and other allergic conditions may be highly associated with eczema.[19] Food allergy complicates eczema treatment and management since exposure to offending foods may cause flares and exacerbations. It is also worth noting from the clinical and laboratory observational studies that TCM therapy for eczema also resulted in reduction of food specific IgE.[3] In this article, we have reviewed published literatures from PubMed and abstract conference presentations selected from studies relevant to TCM for food allergy and eczema.

Results

TCM Formula for FA

Investigational New Drug Derived from TCM

FAHF-2 development: FAHF-2 is the first US FDA botanical investigational new drug (IND) for FA. It was developed from a classic 10-herb formula, Wu Mei Wan, used to treat intestinal parasite infections and gastrointestinal disorders with symptoms similar to FA and gastroenteritis. Ling Zhi (*Ganoderma Lucidum*), an herb with significant anti-inflammatory and anti-allergy effects, was added. This 11-herb formula was named Food Allergy Herbal Formula-1 (FAHF-1). Two herbs, Xi Xin (*Herba cum radice asari*) and Zhi Fu Zi (*Radix lateralis aconiti carmichaeli praeparata*), potentially toxic if improperly processed, were removed. The final 9-herb formula was named FA herbal formula-2 (FAHF-2). The herbal constituents (shown in Fig. 3.1) have long histories in Asian countries and are sold in the US as dietary supplements. Some studies demonstrate benefits of Wu Mei Wan with or without modification on diseases including rash, gastroenteritis, and asthma. No adverse effects were reported. The major preclinical and clinical studies related to FAHF-2, among others natural products, are summarized in Table 3.1.

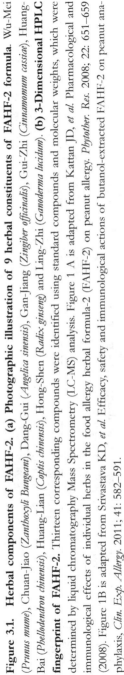

(b)

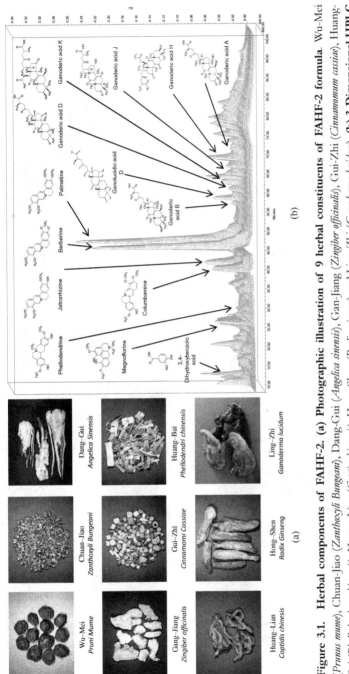

(a)

Figure 3.1. Herbal components of FAHF-2. (a) Photographic illustration of 9 herbal constituents of FAHF-2 formula. Wu-Mei (*Prunus mume*), Chuan-Jiao (*Zanthoxyli Bungeani*), Dang-Gui (*Angelica sinensis*), Gan-Jiang (*Zingiber officinalis*), Gui-Zhi (*Cinnamomum cassiae*), Huang-Bai (*Phellodendron chinensis*), Huang-Lian (*Coptis chinensis*), Hong-Shen (*Radix ginseng*) and Ling-Zhi (*Ganoderma lucidum*). **(b) 3-Dimensional HPLC fingerprint of FAHF-2.** Thirteen corresponding compounds were identified using standard compounds and molecular weights, which were determined by liquid chromatography Mass Spectrometry (LC-MS) analysis. Figure 1 A is adapted from Kattan JD, *et al.* Pharmacological and immunological effects of individual herbs in the food allergy herbal formula-2 (FAHF-2) on peanut allergy. *Phytother. Res.* 2008; 22: 651–659 (2008). Figure 1B is adapted from Srivastava KD, *et al.* Efficacy, safety and immunological actions of butanol-extracted FAHF-2 on peanut anaphylaxis, *Clin. Exp. Allergy.* 2011; 41: 582–591.

Table 3.1.   Summary of TCM therapy for food allergy. Latest treatment including TCM formulas and active compounds, related animal models, clinical trials, and mechanism studies are summarized.

Treatment	Animal Model	Clinical Trials / Human Cells	Mechanisms of Actions
FAHF-2	• Completely prevents PN anaphylaxis and histamine release[20] • Suppressed peanut-specific IgE and Th2 cytokine (IL-5 and IL-13) productions, and increased peanut-specific IgG2a levels and interferon-gamma (IFN-γ) production[21] • Prolongs post-treatment protection against PN anaphylaxis[21]	• Acute and extended phase I trials showed long-term safety and tolerability[24] • Phase II clinical trial showed significant reduction in basophil activation markers in response to ex vivo stimulation at 6 months[25] • Reduction of IL-5 and induction of IL-10 and Tregs in allergen stimulated PBMC cultures[25]	• Blocks vascular leakage associated with anaphylaxis[20] • Inhibits IgE production by human B cells[21] • Exhibits long-lasting beneficial effects on T cells and B cells in vivo[25]
B-FAHF-2	• Protects mice from anaphylaxis induced by PN[49] • Full protection persists up to 8 months post therapy[49] • Additional and longer protection with OIT on tree nuts[50]	• NA	• Dose dependent inhibition of IgE production by human B cells and inhibition of MCs[49] • In vitro suppression of PN-induced Th2 cytokine secretion and enhancement of Th1 cytokine secretion[49]
E-B-FAHF-2	• Protection of peanut-allergic mice from anaphylaxis to peanut challenge[27] • Decrease in peanut specific-IgE in treated mice by approximately 70%[27] • Modulate gut microbiome	• Phase II trial is ongoing, a combination including E-B-FAHF-2 or placebo, multiple OIT to 3 food allergens, and a 4-month course of omalizumab	• In vitro inhibition of IgE production by human B cells in a non-toxic dose-dependent manner[51] • Significantly reduced TNF-α levels in a dose-dependent manner in murine macrophage cells[51]

Formula-3	• Significantly reduced tissue damage in the small intestines, and suppressed Th2 cytokine secretion and IgE production[52] • Significantly suppressed FceR1-mediated mast cell degranulation in OVA-challenged allergic rats[52] • Ameliorate food allergy through modulating the bacterial dysbiosis[53]	• NA • Stabilized mast cells by suppressing FceR1-induced Ca^{2+} mobilization mainly through inhibiting Ca^{2+} entry via store-operated calcium channels[52] • Modules involved in phosphotransferase system and lipopolysaccharide biosynthesis were enriched in FA mice, while Formula-3 treatment enriched pathways of multiple transport system[53]
Combined TCM Regimen for FSFA	• NA • Practice-based evidence study described three pediatric patients with frequent FSFA experienced dramatic reductions in, or elimination of onset[28]	• Prospective study of TCM protective effect on FSFA is underway
Kakkonto	• Significantly suppressed the occurrence of allergic diarrhea and myeloperoxidase activity in the OVA mice[29] • Significantly enhanced the effectiveness of OIT on the allergic symptoms, and the combination therapy further suppresses the Th2 immune responses and the mast cell degranulation[30]	• NA • Reduced mRNA expression of helper T cell type 1 (Th1) cytokines (IFN-gamma), Th2 cytokines (IL-4, IL-5 and IL-10), and suppressor of cytokine signaling-3[29] • Significantly reduced the proportion of CD69+ cells and the elevates helper T cell type 2-specific transcription factor GATA-3 mRNA expression in the LP CD4+ T cells[29]

(Continued)

Table 3.1. (*Continued*)

Treatment	Animal Model	Clinical Trials / Human Cells	Mechanisms of Actions
			• Number of Foxp3-positive cells is dramatically increased in the colonic mucosa of treated FA mice[30] • Increased OIT induced population of Foxp3+ CD4+ regulatory T cells in the FA mouse colon[30] • Reduced the expression of CYP26B1 mRNA in the FA mouse colon[30]
Yokukansan	• NA	• Effective in controlling refractory chronic urticaria[54]	• Inhibited secretion of β-hexosaminidase, intracellular calcium influx, production of TNF-α and ICAM-1 expression[54] • Suppress ICAM-1 expression on human microvascular endothelial cells[54] Inhibits IgE production by Human B cells[26]
Berberine	• Induced long-term tolerance to peanut accompanied by profound and sustained reduction of IgE in peanut-allergic mice	• Inhibits IgE production by PBMCs from patients with FA • Significantly inhibited RBL-2H3 cell and human mast cell degranulation in a non-toxic, dose-dependent manner	• Inhibition IgE production is associated with suppression of epsilon germline transcript (εGLT) expression by PBMCs, a key mechanism that promotes IgE isotype switching[26]

	• Gut bacterial genera positively correlated with post-challenge histamine and PN-IgE included Lachnospiraceae, Ruminococcaceae and Hydrogenanaerobacterium while Verrucromicrobiacea. Caproiciproducens, Enterobacteriaceae and Bacteroidales, were negatively correlated[31]		• Inhibit Xbp1 and STAT6, the critical transcription factor for developing and maintaining long-lived IgE plasma cells • Suppressing effect on spleen tyrosine kinase phosphorylation, which is an IgE- mediated FceRI early signaling event required for degranulation
7,4′-dihydroxyflavone	• In a murine model of allergic asthma, not only significantly reduces eosinophilic pulmonary inflammation, serum IgE levels, IL-4 and IL-13 levels, but also increases IFN-γ production in lung cell cultures in response to antigen stimulation[55]	• NA	• Inhibited Th2 memory cells IL-4, IL-5, IL- 13 production by inhibition of GATA3 expression[55] • Significantly inhibited Dex long term culture augmentation of p-STAT6 and impaired HDAC2 expression and Dex increased eotaxin production [56] • Significantly reduced IL-8 production by human colon epithelial cells, associated with reduction of phosphorylated IxBα[51]
Ganoderic acid C1	• NA	• Inhibited TNF-α production by PBMCs from patients with allergies or Crohn's disease [57]	• Inhibited TNF-α production by macrophage cell line • Inhibition of TNF-α production is mediated by down-regulation of NFxB, MAPK, and AP-1

(Continued)

Table 3.1. (*Continued*)

Treatment	Animal Model	Clinical Trials / Human Cells	Mechanisms of Actions
Ganoderic acid B	• NA	• Inhibited TNF-α, IL-6 production by PBMCs from patients with allergies • Increased IL-10, IL-12, and IFN-γ production by PBMCs from patients with allergies.	• Inhibited TNF-α production by macrophage cell line [58]
Formonon etin	• NA	• Significantly decreased IgE production in human B cells, without cytotoxicity[59]	• Inhibited STAT6, NF-kB phosphorylation, as well as Xbp1 and IgE heavy chain expression
Xanthopur purin	• Significantly reduced anaphylaxis scores of peanut allergic mice in both early and late treatment experiments, associated with significant reduction of plasma histamine levels • Reduced peanut-specific IgE levels by 80% (p<0.01), associated with significant reduction of IL-4 without affecting IgG, IgA, or IFN-g production. • Strong post-therapy protection at least 5 weeks after the treatment[60]	• Significantly and dose-dependently inhibited IgE production in human B cell line and PBMCs from food allergic subjects	• Reduced peripheral and bone marrow IgE+B cells compared to the untreated group • XBP-1 was identified as one of the important transcription factors associated with XPP suppression of IgE

Preclinical study of FAHF-2: Using an established murine peanut-allergy model, FAHF-2 significantly protected mice from anaphylaxis when orally challenged with peanut.[20] This was associated with suppressed peanut-specific IgE and Th2 cytokines (IL-5 and IL-13), enhanced peanut-specific IgG2a levels, and increased IFN-γ production. Effects persisted 6 months post treatment — 25 % of life-span.[21] B cells and T cells were modulated, and basophil and mast-cell activation was suppressed directly by suppressing IgE-induced FcεRI expression, contributing to long-term protection.[22] Mice fed 24 times effective daily dose showed no signs of toxicity, abnormal liver and kidney function, or abnormal CBC or major organ histology.[20]

Clinical study of FAHF-2 (phase I and II trials): Given its efficacy and safety in the murine model, the U.S. FDA approved it as an IND (No. 77,468) in 2007. The first human study was a phase I trial investigating safety — the first US clinical safety trial of TCM for FA.[23] Eighteen subjects allergic to peanut, tree nut, fish, and/or shellfish were enrolled in this double-blind, placebo-controlled dose escalation trial, receiving 4, 6, or 12 tablets three times a day for 7 days. Doses were well-tolerated, and no significant observed adverse effects. The FAHF-2 group showed suppressed IL-5 and increases in IFN-γ. Long-term safety and tolerability were assessed in an open label extended phase II trial. Subjects received six tablets three times a day for 6 months. FAHF-2 was well-tolerated and significantly suppressed basophil activation.[24]

The phase II clinical trial was double-blind, placebo-controlled. Subjects 12 to 45 years, allergic to peanut, tree nut, sesame, fish or shellfish, were recruited. FAHF-2 or placebo treatment was 10 tablets three times daily for 6 months. The primary outcome was change in reaction threshold during oral food challenge before and after treatment. Sixty-eight subjects were enrolled at 3 US sites. Treatment was well-tolerated with no serious adverse events. In vitro studies of the peripheral blood mononuclear cells (PBMCs) culture showed significantly suppressed IL-5 and induction of IL-10 and Tregs, indicating immune cells exposed to sufficient FAHF-2 switched from an allergic to a non-allergic phenotype.[25] However, the primary endpoint was not met, perhaps due to poor adherence in 44% of subjects.

Development of B-FAHF-2 and EB-FAHF-2: A major drawback was high daily dosage. Therefore, FAHF-2 using butanol purification — B-FAHF-2

(BF2) — was developed, concentrating active compounds by removing non-medicinal compounds. In vitro study in IgE-producing human plasma cell line showed that BF2 was 9 times more potent than FAHF-2 in suppressing IgE, and that BF2 at ~1/5 the dose of FAHF-2 protected from peanut anaphylaxis in the murine model.[26] In a peanut/tree nut allergy murine model, BF2 plus OIT with peanut and multiple nuts treated mice experienced fewer, milder adverse reactions than OIT-only (p<0.01) during the one-day rush OIT buildup. They showed greater, more persistent protection against challenge 5-6 weeks post-therapy. BF2+OIT mediated protection was associated with significantly lower plasma histamine and IgE levels, higher IFN-γ /IL-4 and IL-10/ IL-4 ratios, DNA remethylation at IL-4 promoter and demethylation at IFN-g and Foxp3 promoters. Challenge symptom scores were inversely correlated with IL-4 DNA methylation.

In moving BF2 to clinical studies, large-scale extraction of Ling Zhi proved difficult, so ethyl acetate, a solvent used to decaffeinate coffee and tea, was employed. The enhanced formula — E-B-FAHF-2 (EBF2) — inhibited in vitro plasma cell line IgE production in a non-toxic dose-dependent manner much more potently than its precursors. Across three separate in vivo experiments, EBF2 completely protected peanut-allergic mice from anaphylaxis. Peanut specific-IgE fell 70%.[27] EBF2 IgE inhibition was associated with IgE heavy chain suppression.

Phase II clinical study of EBF2: The FDA has approved study of combined EBF2, multi OIT, and Xolair (Omalizumab) for FA. The trial includes EBF2 or placebo (max 4 capsules twice daily), multiple OIT to 3 food allergens, and 4-month course of omalizumab. Primary outcome is sustained unresponsiveness to all three allergens after 2 years. The trial is ongoing in two sites in the US.

Practice Based Evidence Study: Combined TCM Regimen for Frequent and Severe Food Anaphylaxis

Despite strict avoidance, some severely food-allergic children experience frequent severe food anaphylaxis (FSFA) triggered by skin contact or inhalation, leading to numerous emergency room visits and ICU admissions. A practice-based evidence (real-life) study described successful prevention of FSFA by combined TCM regimen.[28] Three patients ages 9–16 years (P1 allergic to milk; P2 and P3 to tree nuts) were analyzed. All experienced numerous reactions (30–400), requiring rescue medications (5–50 time) and emergency room visits (5–40 time) during the 2 years prior to TCM. Modified Pruni Mume Formula (Remedy A), Fructus Jujubae Formula (Remedy B), a Phellodendron chinensis containing herbal bath additive (Remedy C), and herbal cream (Remedy D) were provided. These children experienced dramatic reductions or elimination of FSFA.

Such practice-based evidence studies may provide a new approach to investigate the efficacy of TCM for specific patient groups more quickly than randomized controlled trials. In 2018, FDA began to accept real-world study data. Given TCM's nature as personalized medicine, this new mechanism may facilitate clinical study of botanical medicine.

Japanese-Chinese Traditional Medicine Kakkonto

Japanese traditional medicine, Kampo, derived in antiquity from Chinese medicine, shares TCM concepts and herbs. There are several studies about the herbal formula Kakkonto for FA. Using an OVA-induced intestinal food allergic model, oral Kakkonto was shown to significantly suppress allergic diarrhea and myeloperoxidase activity, associated with modulation on Th1, Th2, and Tregs.[29] Kakkonto showed beneficial effects by enhancing Th2 inhibition and Treg enhancement.[30] Kakkonto could reduce mRNA expression of helper T cell type 1 (Th1) cytokines (IFN-γ), Th2 cytokines (IL-4, IL-5 and IL-10), and suppressing cytokine signaling-3.

Active TCM Compounds for Treating FA

FAHF-2 and its refined successors have shown sustainable suppression of IgE and mast cell/basophil activation, and modulated cytokine profiles. We have begun to identify active compounds that target specific mechanisms and established a natural product library to identify anti-FA active compounds. Major findings are summarized below.

Berberine, the most abundant major ingredient in FAHF-2, was isolated from *Philodendron chinensis*. It potently inhibits IgE production by PBMCs in FA patients, with an IC50 value as low as 0.1962 (μg/mL). Berberine suppressed epsilon germline transcript (εGLT) expression by PBMCs, a key mechanism for IgE isotype switching.[26] A recent study showed berberine inhibited Xbp1 and STAT6, the critical transcription factor for developing and maintaining long-lived IgE plasma cells.[9]

Berberine significantly inhibited rodent and human mast cell degranulation in a non-toxic, dose-dependent manner. It showed suppression of spleen tyrosine kinase (Syk) phosphorylation, an IgE-mediated FcεRI early signaling event for degranulation,[22] suggesting value for FA and other mast cell disorders.

Recently we evaluated an orally available BBR-containing natural medicine (BCNM) as FA treatment and explored whether treatment-induced gut microbiota changes correlated with therapeutic outcomes. The results showed that BCNM-treatment regimen induced long-term peanut tolerance with profound, sustained IgE reduction in murine model of peanut allergy. Significant differences were observed for Firmicutes/Bacteroidetes ratio. Bacterial genera positively correlated with post-challenge histamine and peanut-IgE included Lachnospiraceae, Ruminococcaceae, and Hydrogenanaerobacterium, while Verrucromicrobiacea, Caproiciproducens, Enterobacteriaceae, and Bacteroidales were negatively correlated.[31] So BCNM is effective as FA treatment and has benefits associated with a distinct microbiota signature in mice.

Moreover, active compounds including 7,4′-dihydroxyflavone (7,4′-DHF), ganoderic C1 (GAC1), ganoderic β (GAβ), formononetin, and xanthopurpurin are also proven to show excellent anti-allergy activities. The detailed efficacy and mechanisms are listed in Table 1. The results suggest that 7,4′-DHF (isolated from *glycyrrhiza uralensis*), GAC1, and GAβ (isolated from *ganoderma lucidum*) have the potential to treat both IgE-mediated and non-IgE-mediated FA and other inflammatory conditions. In addition, formononetin (isolated from *sophora flavescens*) and xanthopurpurin (isolated from *rubia cordifolia*) may apply on IgE-mediated FA and other allergic conditions.

In summary, TCM for FA has gone through several phases. First was to adapt a traditional formulation for conditions such as parasite infection and GI symptoms (FAHF2). Laboratory and preliminary clinical studies demonstrated safety and preliminary efficacy. Second, purifying to increase potency and facilitate adherence (B-FAHF2 and EB-FAHF2). Finally, state-of-the-art technology was used to identify pure active compounds (FAHF-2 and other potential natural product libraries). These phases provided knowledge to develop bioavailability, potency, and precision (targeting memory IgE and inflammatory response) to fundamentally alter both IgE-mediated and non-IgE mediated FA as novel botanical medicines.

TCM Formula for Eczema

Efficacy Analysis for Clinical Study of TCM in Treating Eczema

Triple TCM Therapy

It is believed that eczema treatment can be enhanced with a multifaceted approach. Thus, concurrent topical and oral TCM treatments are being used to relieve discomfort, correct internal and external immune disorders, and improve skin barrier function. Our group has developed several TCM therapy approaches for eczema that include herbal internal supplements, additives, and creams/ointments (remedies A–C). These aim to relieve excessive itching, inhibit microbial infection, and reduce inflammatory reactions. Shi Zhen Tea I is derived from the textbook — *Practical Diagnostic and Therapeutics and Integrated Traditional Chinese and Western Medicine.*[32] And Shi Zhen Tea Ia is modified from traditional Xiao Feng San, where *schizonepta stem, burdock fruit, atractylodes rhizome,* and *shrubby sophora root* are reserved as main herbs against inflammation and microorganism, while *cicada molting* and *silkworm* can be used to relieve itching. Table 3.2 summarizes the herbal constituents of each of these remedies in ingested and topical TCM formulations for different disease stages. For example, Cream I (Lo/la) and Herbal Bath Additive plus Supplement I is used for acute and severe eczema. Supplement Ia can be added to relieve excessive itching and when antihistamines fail. During dose and frequency reduction and maintenance when eczema is well-controlled, Cream II, Herbal Bath Additive, and Supplement I or II are used until stopping treatment. Modifications are allowed in considering individual's additional conditions. The pharmacological effects and mechanisms of actions of key herbal constituents are summarized in Table 3.4. Treatment of moderate-to-severe eczema with this combined regimen was studied in several clinical retrospective analyses.[33,34]

Table 3.2.   Clinical research of TCM formulas on the treatment for eczema. Eight sets of TCM clinical therapies with 10 clinical trials for the treatment of eczema are introduced.

Formula Name	Herb Constituents	Usage and Function	Clinical Researched Outcomes
Triple TCM Therapy: Remedy A (Forsythia formula/Shi Zhen Tea I/Supplement I)	Fu Ling (*Poria sclerotium*) Dan Pi (*Tree peony root bark*) Di Fu Zi (*Summer cypress fruit*) Jin Yin Hua (*Honeysuckle flower bud*) Zi Cao (*Red-root lithospermum root*) Lian Qiao (*Forsythia Fruit*) Qing Dai (Boil wrapped) (*Indigo dye extract from leaf*) Sheng Gan Cao (*Chinese licorice root & rhizome*)	• As dietary supplement • For acute eczema with redness, itching, woozy, and rash • Reduce systemic inflammation and improve gut function • Antimicrobial	**Study 1**[33]: 14 patients, including 9 male and 5 female patients, with moderate-to-severe AD [median age 5.4 yrs (IQR 0.5–52)] • Significant improvements in both disease severity (SCORAD) and quality of life (DLQI) of patients • Significant reduction in topical steroid, antibiotics, and antihistamines use of patients after 3 months of TCM • A statistically significant decrease in peanut-specific IgE • Increase skin integrity and promote skin regeneration>reduce infection
Remedy A1 (Burdock Fruit/Shi Zhen Tea1a/Supplement1a)	Jing Jie (*Schizonepeta Stem*) Niu Bang Zi (*Burdock Fruit*) Bai Zhu (*Atractylodes Rhizome*) Ku Shen (*Shrubby sophora root*) Chan Tui (*Cicada Molting*) Jiang Can (*Silkworm*)	• As dietary supplement • For chronic eczema • For individuals with excessive itching • Antihistamine/microbial	**Study 2**[36]: 28 patients with eczema divided into three cohorts based on eczema phenotype/endotype • Cohort #1 (n=10), ages 6 to 48 months, with moderate to severe eczema. TCM reduced SCORAD and steroid use as early as one month (p<0.001) and close to zero by 6 months • Cohort #2 (n=8), ages 2–40 years, had severe eczema associated with sudden topical steroid withdrawal (TSW, n=8) at least 3 months prior to TCM. TCM showed improved SCORAD (73.6%,

Remedy	Herbs	Functions	Clinical results
Remedy B Phellodendron Herbal Bath I	Huang Bo (*Phellodendron bark*) Da Huang (*Chinese rhubarb*) Bai Xian Pi (*Dictamnus root bark*) Bai Ji Li (*Tribulus fruit*) Ku Shen (*Shrubby sophora*) Tu Fu Ling (*Chinese smilax rhizome*)	• External treatments for Remedy A, F or G • Washed daily with the herbal bath • For acute eczema • Reduce skin local inflammation and improvement skin itching integrity, keep hydration • Antimicrobial	$p < 0.001$), and markedly decreased sleep disturbance (80%, $p < 0.001$) as early as one month • Cohort #3 had a very high total IgE (>5,000 kIU/L, n=10), ages 1–13 years. Cohort #3 had markedly reduced total IgE from median 12,328 to 3,994 kIU/L and reduced elevated blood eosinophils ($p < 0.05$) after 6–24 months
Remedy C (Indigo Herbal Cream I [Cream Lo/La])	Bai Ji Li (*Tribulus fruit*) Dang Gui (*Angelica Root*) Jin Yin Hua (*Honeysuckle Flower*) Zi Cao (hong) (*Lithospermum Root*) Ku Shen (*Shrubby sophora*) Qing Dai (*Indigo (Isatis) Leaf Extract*) Bing Pian (*Borneol*)	• External treatments for • For acute and most severe phase • Reduce skin local inflammation and improvement in skin integrity, keep hydration • Antimicrobial	
Remedy C2 (Phellodendron /Herbal Cream II)	Huang Bo (*Phellodendron chinensis*) Qing Dai (*Indigo extract from leaf*)	• External treatments • For the recovering phase • Reduce skin local inflammation, protect recovered skin, and improvement of skin integrity and barrier	

(*Continued*)

Table 3.2. *(Continued)*

Formula Name	Herb Constituents	Usage and Function	Clinical Researched Outcomes
Xiao Feng San[61]	Fang Feng (*Saposhnikovia divaricate*) Jing Jie (*Schizonepeta tenuifolia*) Dang Gui (*Angelica sinensis*) Di Huang (*Rehmannia glutinosa*) Ku Shen (*Sophora flavescens*) Cang Zhu (*Atractylodes lancea*) Chan Tui (*Cryptotympana pustulata*) Ya Ma (*Linum usitatissimum*) Zhi Mu (*Anemarrhena asphodeloides*) Shi Gao (*Gypsum fibrosum*) Mu Tong (*Clematis armandii*) Gan Cao (*Glycyrrhiza uralensis*) Niu Bang Zi (*Arctium lappa*)	• As dietary supplement • Relieve itching and pain, anti-inflammatory, harmonizes water metabolism, sedative, protects digestive system, and antibacterial	**Study 3**[61]: 71 patients with severe intractable atopic dermatitis into two group for 8-week treatment: XFS (47 patients) or placebo (24 patients) • A significant improvement in XFS group in erythema, surface damage, pruritus, and sleep • No statistical differences in immunologic makers (e.g., IL-5, IL-13, IgE, eosinophil count, eosinophil cationic protein) between XFS and placebo groups during an 8-week treatment period
Pei Tu Qing Xin Tang (PTQXT)[38]	Tai Zi; Chen (*Radix Pseudostellariae*) Lian Qiao (*Forsythia suspense*) Gou Teng (*Ramulus Uncariae cum Uncis*) Deng Xin Cao (*Medulla Junci*) Dan Zhu Ye (*Herba Lophatheri*) Yi Yi Ren (*Semen Coicis*)	• As dietary supplement • Invigorate the spleen and reduce dampness, clear heart-fire, and relieve itching • Reinforcing the immune function and regulating the digestive function	**Study 4**[38]: 250 patients with moderate-to- severe eczema were divided into three groups: A (oral administration of PTQXT), B (oral administration of PTQXT and external wash formula), and C (positive control with mometasne furoate) • Lesser disease severity and improved QOL and patients' self-assessment were observed during the treatment for all groups

	Shan Yao (*Rhizoma Dioscoreae*) Mu Li (*Concha Ostreae*) Gan Cao (*Radix Glycyrrhizae*) Shui Niu Jiao (*Cornu Bubali*) Fu Ling (*Poria*) Bai Zhu (*Rhizoma Atractylodis Macrocephalae*)	• Antimicrobial, anti-inflammatory, anti-oxidative	• The SCORAD in both TCM groups was significantly lower than that in the control group in the follow-up period • The QOL and the patients' self- assessment in both TCM groups were better than that in the control group in the follow-up period • All patients had normal renal and liver function
Wash formula with PTQXT[58]	Jin Yin Hua (*Flos Lonicerae*) Huang Jing (*Rhizoma Polygonati*) Bo He (*Herba Menthae*) Gan Cao (*Radix Glycyrrhizae*)	• External treatments with PTQXT • Washed skin • Good antibacterial activities, especially against *Staphylococcus aureus*	
Pentaherbs Formula[39, 40]	Jin Yin Hua (*Flos Lonicerae*) Bo He (*Herba menthae*) Dan Pi (*Cortex moutan*) Cang Zhu (*Rhizoma atractylodis*) Huang Bo (*Cortex phellodendri*)	• As dietary supplement • Reducing topical corticosteroid usage in children with moderate-to-severe atopic dermatitis	**Study 5**[39]: 85 patients were divided into TCM and placebo groups • The SCORADs decreased during the study period for two groups with no significant difference • The duration and quantity of corticosteroid (mometasone furoate) usage in the TCM group was significantly reduced but not in placebo group • No derangement in haematological or biochemical parameters during treatment **Study 6**[40]: 22 children (4–7 years) with moderate-to-severe AD • The syrup significantly improves AD severity and quality of life

(Continued)

Table 3.2.   (*Continued*)

Formula Name	Herb Constituents	Usage and Function	Clinical Researched Outcomes
Hochuekki- to (known as BZYQT[62] in China, and Bojungikki-tang in Korea)	Ren Shen (*Ginseng radix*) Cang Zhu (*Atractylodis rhizome*) Huang Qi (*Astragali radix*) Dang Gui (*Angelicae radix*) Da Zao (*Ziziphi fructus*) Chai Hu (*Bupleuri radix*) Gan Cao (*Glycyrrhizae radix*) Sheng Jiang (*Zingiberis rhizome*) Sheng Ma (*Cimicifugae rhizome*) Chen Pi (*Aurantii nobilis Pericarpium*)	• As dietary supplement. • Correcting abnormal homeostasis of the body and regulating immune function • Alleviate *Kikyo* (delicate, easily fatigable or hypersensitive) of patients with atopic dermatitis	• Hematological and biochemical profiles remained within normal limits during the treatment phase **Study 7**[62]: 84 patients with Kikyo constitution were divided into two groups: *Hochu-ekki-to* group and placebo group • The administration of *Hochu-ekki-to* significantly reduces dosage of topical steroids and/or tacrolimus, compared with placebo • The post-treatment prominent efficacy rate tends to be higher in the *Hochu-ekki- to* group than in the placebo group
Qin-Zhu-Liang-Xue deoction[42]	Fang Feng (*Saposhnikovia divaricate*) Gan Cao (*Glycyrrhiza uralensis Fisch.*) Huang Qin (*Scutellaria baicalensis Georgi*) Mu Dan Pi (*Paeonia suffruticosa Andr.*)	• As dietary supplement • Enhance both innate and adaptive immunity • Alleviating symptoms of atopic eczema, maintaining long-term stability, and improving patient quality of life	**Study 8**[42]: 168 patients were divided into QZLX group (treatment group) and Run- Zao-Zhi-Yang (RZZY) groups (control group). • QZLXD was potentially safe and more effective than RZZYC in treating sub- acute eczema of blood-heat type • QZLXD is effective in relieving symptoms of eczema, reducing relapse rates, and enhancing the itching threshold of histamine phosphate

Yi Yi Ren (*Coix lacryma-jobi L. var. mayuen*) Mu Li (*Ostrea gigas Thimberg*) Zhen Zhu Mu (*Hyriopsis cumingii*) Ci Shi (*Magnetite*) Zi Cao (*Arnebia euchroma*)		
Jaungo Herbal ointment[43] Zi Cao (*Lithospermi radix*) Dang Gui (*Angelica gigantis radix*) *sesame seed oil bees wax swine oil*	• For xerosis cutis, frostbite, miliaria, anal fissures, and rhus dermatitis and approved by Korea Food and Drug Administration • Applied to affected skin areas • Antibacterial, anti-inflammatory, antioxidant, regeneration-promoting, and moisturizing effects	**Study 9**[43]: 34 patients with mild-to- moderate AD were divided into three group: treatment 1 (applies Jaungo twice a day), treatment 2 (applies Jaungo and placebo ointments once a day), and placebo group (applies placebo ointment twice a day) • Jaungo is effective for the treatment of AD, especially for chronic phase symptoms such as excoriation, lichenification, and dryness • Both the excoriation and lichenification scores in the EASI decreased significantly in treatment group 1 indicating that Jaungo had the effect of wound healing
Multiple component TCM[44] *(Formula I)* Ku Shen (*Sophora flavescens*) Hu Zhang (*Polygonum cuspidatum*) Da Qing Ye (*Isatis tinctoria*) Tu Fu Ling (*Smilax glabra*) Dang Gui (*Angelica dahurica*)	• As dietary supplement. • Anti-inflammatory, antimicrobial, anti- oxidative	**Study 10**[44]: 94 patients suffering from severe and/or intractable forms of the AD were treated by multiple components TCM including formula I, lotion II, and ointment III for 3 years.

(Continued)

Table 3.2. *(Continued)*

Formula Name	Herb Constituents	Usage and Function	Clinical Researched Outcomes
	Gan Cao (*Glycyrrhiza uralensis*) Huang Qin (*Scutellaria baicalensis*) Ju Hua (*Chrysanthemum indicum*) Xia Ku Cao (*Prunella vulgaris*) Bai Hua She She Cao (*Oldenlandia diffusa*)		• The TCM treatment markedly improved the atopic symptoms of AD with a significant reduction in clinical AD severity score and pruritus score, leading to an effective rate as good as 97% • EOS in white blood cell differentiation and serum IgE levels, which displayed a statistically significant decrease • No obvious abnormalities could be detected in any study participant
Multiple component TCM[44] *(Lotion II)*	Ku Shen (*Sophora flavescens*) Huang Lian (*Coptis chinensis*) Huang Qin (*Scutellaria baicalensis*) Bai Bu (*Stemona sessilifolia*) Shi Liu Pi (*Punica granatum*) Ju Hua (*Chrysanthemum indicum*) Qi Ye Yi Zhi Hua (*Paris polyphylla*)	• External treatments for formula I • Washed daily with the concentrated aqueous lotion • Contribution to the dry skin going with rushes and other forms of skin irritation	
Multiple component TCM[44] *(Ointment III)*	Ku Shen (*Sophora flavescens*) Hu Zhang (*Polygonum cuspidatum*) Da Qing Ye (*Isatis tinctoria*) Dang Gui (*Angelica dahurica*) Gan Cao (*Glycyrrhiza uralensis*) Huang Qin (*Scutellaria baicalensis*)	• External treatments for formula I • Applied to all affected skin areas • Contribution to the dry skin going with rushes and other forms of skin irritation	

Triple TCM Therapy for Recalcitrant Eczema

While the treatment of eczema is well documented in TCM literature,[35] studies on its effect on corticosteroid-refractory eczema is limited. A recent retrospective analysis from our group by Thanik *et al.*[33] (Study 1, Table 2) reported therapeutic effects of TCM on skin lesions and quality of life. The study included 14 patients (13 children, 1 adult), median age 5.4 years (interquartile range [IQR], 0.5–52 years). In addition to daily topical steroids, half reported using oral corticosteroids. 13 of the 14 were defined as severe disease based on SCORing Atopic Dermatitis (SCORAD score >50). Following TCM treatment at a median of 8 months (range, 3–24 months), SCORAD was significantly reduced from baseline score 89 (range, 42–103) to post therapy 1 (range, 0–62; $P < .001$, Fig. 2A). Median Dermatology Life Quality Index (DLQI) scores were also significantly reduced from baseline of 17 (range, 10–30) to 1 (range, 0–14; $P < .0001$, Fig. 2B, Fig. 2C–G) post therapy. Furthermore, 69% reported stopping use of topical steroids, 80% stopped oral steroids, and 80% stopped using antihistamines. The cyclosporine patient discontinued it after 3 months of TCM. All 9 patients using antibiotics for *Staphylococcus aureus* superinfection at onset of TCM treatment discontinued antibiotics, and no superinfections occurred during treatment.

Triple TCM Therapy for Eczema Patients with Features of Steroid Dependent, Steroid Withdrawal, Laboratory High IgE Levels, And Eosinophils

In this study, 28 patients with moderate-to-severe eczema were divided into 3 cohorts based on eczema phenotype/endotype (abstract published by Yang *et al.*).[36] In Cohort #1 (n=10) — infants and young children (ages 6 to 48 months) with moderate to severe eczema — 8 of them used topical steroids for at least 3 months prior to TCM. Cohort #2 (n=8), ages 2–40 years, had worsening eczema associated with sudden topical steroid withdrawal (TSW, n=8) at least 3 months prior to TCM. Cohort #3 had a very high total IgE (>5,000 kIU/L, n=6), ages 1–13 years. Following treatment, cohort #1 showed reduced SCORAD, and steroid use as early as one month (p<0.001); close to zero by 6 months (Fig. 3). Cohort #2 showed improved SCORAD (73.6%, p<0.001), and markedly decreased sleep disturbance (80%, p<0.001)

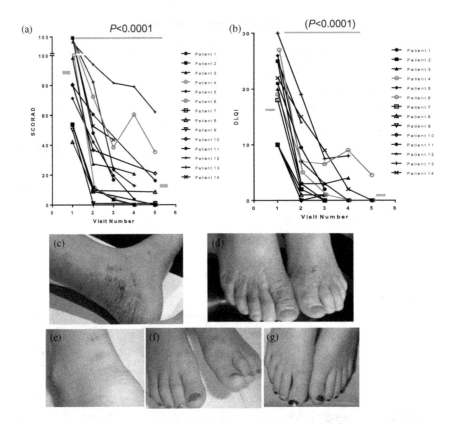

Figure 3.2. A. Effect of Triple TCM Therapy on AD severity Scores: (a) SCORing Atopic Dermatitis (SCORAD) from onset of TCM treatment (visit 1) through a median follow-up of 8 (IQR 3-24) months of treatment (visit 2-5). **(b)** Effect of Triple TCM Therapy on Dermatology Life Quality Index (DLQI) Scores before and after TCM from onset of TCM treatment (visit 1) through 5 (IQR 3-24) months of treatment (visit 2-5). N=14. ****$P<0.0001$ vs baseline. **(c) Photographs of patient 6.** (c-d) Start of TCM; (e) 6 months; (f) 8 month; and (g) 14 months after TCM. The blue color on the skin is from herbal cream. No topical steroid was used during the period of TCM treatment time. Fig 2(c–g) are adapted from Thanik *et al.* Improvement of skin lesions and life quality in moderate-to-severe eczema patients by combined TCM therapy. Ann Allergy Asthma Immunol. 2018 Jul;121(1):135–136.3.

as early as one month. Cohort #3 had reduced total IgE from median 12,328 to 3,994 kIU/L after 6–24 months. TCM significantly reduced elevated blood eosinophils (p<0.05). No liver or kidney function abnormalities were observed.

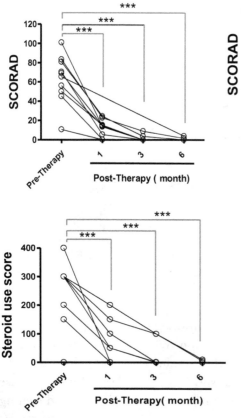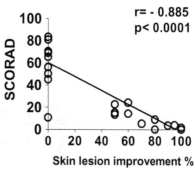

Figure 3.3. **Effect of TCM on infant/early childhood eczema. (a)** Reduction of **SCORAD.** 10 patients ages 6 months to 48 months (median age 16.5-month months) were recruited. Male/female: 6/4. Onset age 0.2 –24 months (median 3 months). SCORAD values were evaluated at the base line (0M) and 1, 3, and 6 months of TCM therapy and showed significant reduction at 1, 3, and 6 of TCM therapy. N = 10. ***p < 0.001 vs baseline. **(b) Correlation analysis of SCORAD and % of Improvement.** At each evaluation, patients' families were asked self-evaluation of skin improvement compared to baseline. There was significant negative correlation between SCORAD and % of improvement by Pearson analysis. R = –0.885, P < 0.0001 (N = 10). **(c) TCM reduced corticosteroid use while improving skin lesion.** Of 10 patients, 7 patients were on topic corticosteroid and 1 on oral corticosteroid at least 3 months prior to TCM. Criteria for Rating Steroid Use Index are as follows: 100 = 1% HC, 2 times per day; 200 = 2.5% HC, 2 times per day; 300 = triamcinolone/Fluticasone, Mometasone Desonide, alclometasone, protopic, 1-2 times per day; 400 = Oral prednisone at least one course/month. There were significant reductions at 1, 3, 6 months of TCM treatment. At 6 months of TCM, steroid use reduced nearly to 0. N = 8*** p < 0.001 vs baseline.

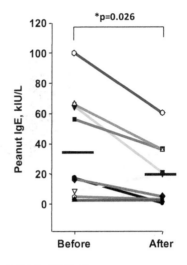

Figure 3.4. A. Effect of Triple TCM Therapy on peanut-specific IgE: Peanut-specific IgE levels before and after TCM therapy after median of 8 months (3-24 months) n = 10. *p < 0.05 vs baseline.

Triple TCM therapy was also demonstrated to reduce peanut-specific IgE (Fig. 4)[33]. This in vitro study demonstrated that remedy A taken as supplement significantly reduced IL-4 production[33] without cytotoxicity, and also reduced eotaxin, TNF-a, and IgE in various cell lines.[36] These studies mechanistically demonstrated a potentially steroid-sparing therapy.

More efficacy and mechanism studies of TCM formula are shown in Table 3.2 including Xiao Feng San (XFS),[37] Pei Tu Qing Xin Tang (PTQXT),[38] PentaHerbs,[39,40] Bu Zhong Yi Qi Tang (BZYQT),[41] Qin Zhu Liang Xue decoction (QZLXD),[42] Jaungo,[43] and A Multiple Component.[44]

Safety Analysis of TCM In Treating Eczema

Our triple therapy was well-tolerated[33] without abnormal liver or kidney function or blood cell counts in the 14-patient cohort (Table 3.3). There were no clinical or laboratory abnormalities in the 28-patient cohort.[36] We studied acute and sub-chronic toxicity of (Remedy A) in animal model (not shown). Mice received oral 5X or 10X treatment doses for 14 days with no mortality or detected morbidity. Cochrane systematic review suggested oral

Table 3.3. Clinical laboratory safety analysis. Copy of laboratory record of complete blood test and liver and kidney fund testing collected from the patient before and after TCM treatment.

Laboratory Value	Pre-treatment Mean (SD)	Post-treatment Mean (SD)	Normal Reference Range
WBC (K/μL)	8.8 ± 3.5; N=9	7.2 ± 2.4; N=10	5–14.5 K/μL
Hemoglobin (g/dL)	13 ± 0.8; N=9	12.5 ± 0.7; N=10	11.5–13.5 g/dL
Platelets (K/μL)	358 ± 115; N=9	323 ± 101; N=9	150–450 K/μL
Urea (mg/dL)	12 ± 4; N=7	12.7 ± 5.8; N=10	7–23 mg/dL
Creatinine (mg/dL)	0.46 ± 0.1 N=7	0.41 ± 0.2; N=11	0.5–1.3 mg/dL
AST (U/L)	33 ± 8; N=5	33 ± 8; N=12	15–46 U/L
ALT (U/L)	34 ± 25; N=5	19 ± 6; N=12	13–69 U/L

use of TCM may improve quality of life for children with moderate or severe atopic eczema and recommended further high-quality studies[35]. No severe adverse events were reported in this and other reviews.[35] Laboratory safety data were not reported. Clinically used TCM is generally safe and well tolerated. Studies are needed on dose response, bioavailability, safety, and efficacy.

Progress in Mechanisms Investigation of Prevailing Top 10 Herbs and Active Compounds in Treating Eczema

Based on the herbal constituents included in the formulas in Table 3.2 and the 10 most-prescribed herbs for treating AD in Taiwan[45], we selected the 10 key herbs and reviewed their mechanisms of action. Names, clinical use, pharmacological effects, and mechanisms are listed in Table 3.4. Most herbs show immunoregulatory, anti-bacterial (*S. aureus, M. tuberculosis, E. coli, T. vaginalis, Amoebaes, Analgesic, S. agalactiae, B. dysenteriae, D. pneumonia, H. streptococcus, C. diphtheria*), and anti-inflammatory effects, preventing infection, restoring barriers, rebalancing Th1/Th2 cells, and regulating cytokine and chemokine production.

With the discovery of biological targets and the development of bioinformatics, computational analysis such as system pharmacology and molecular docking provide us with efficient tools to investigate therapeutic

Table 3.4.　Review of the top 10 herbs and recent publications on mechanism study in relation to eczema. The table includes the name, clinical use, pharmacological effects, and latest mechanism studies.

Chinese Pin Yin Name (Pharmaceutical Name)	TCM Clinical Use	Pharmacological Effects	Mechanism of Action of Herbs and Active Compounds
Gan Cao (Radix Glycyrrhizae)	• Neutral • Sweet • Carbuncles • Bronchitis • Tuberculosis • Peptic ulcers • Frostbite	Relieve pain Immunoregulation Anti-inflammatory Anti-viral Anti-bacterial • S. aureus • M. tuberculosis • E. coli • T. vaginalis	• Hot water extracts of Radix Glycyrrhizae (RG) showed anti-allergic effects on IgE-mediated immediate hypersensitivity in mice.[63] • 18β-Glycyrrhetinic acid from RG, can exert immunomodulatory effects by suppressing Th2 cytokines (IL-5, IL-13) production through upregulation of forkhead box p3 (Foxp3), and downregulation of signal transducer and activator of transcription (STAT6), GATA-binding protein 3 (GATA-3), and retinoic acid-related orphan receptor γt (RORγt) expression.[64]
Ku Shen (Radix Sophorae Flavescentis)	• Cold • Bitter • Dermatological disorders • Chronic bronchitis or bronchial asthma • Insomnia	Kill parasites Relieve Itching Immunostimulant Anti-tumor Anti-viral Anti-bacterial • S. aureus • S. agalactiae • B. dysenteriae • E. coli	• Radix Sophorae Flavescentis (RSF) and RG extracts inhibited production of IL-4 and IL-5 by murine memory Th2 cells and eotaxin-1 production by HLF-1 cells.[65] • The anti-asthma mechanism of modified Ku-Shen-Gan-Cao Formula may be involved in the regulation of the metabolic pathways including fatty acid metabolism, sphingolipid metabolism, glycerophospholipid metabolism, purine metabolism, tryptophan metabolism, bile acid metabolism, and arachidonic acid metabolism.[66]

Herb	Properties & Indications	Anti-bacterial	Pharmacology
Huang Qin (Radix Scutellariae)	• Bitter • Cold • Jaundice and hepatitis • Dysentery • Hypertension Hepatoprotective Anti-inflammatory Anti-viral Anti-tumor Anti-oxidant Anti-bacterial	• *S. aureus* • *D. pneumonia* • *P. aeruginosa*	• The ethanol extracts of *RS* had a significant inhibitory effect on allergic inflammation *in vivo* and *in vitro* by down-regulation of expression of various inflammatory mediators and decreasing the production of inflammatory cytokines and MAPK activation.[67] • Wogonin, an active ingredient of *RS*, could downregulate the OVA-induced Th2 immune response, strongly inhibit the production of IL-5, and indirectly reduce IgE levels without reduction in cell viability.[68]
Dang Gui (Radicis Angelicae Sinensis)	• Sweet • Acrid • Warm • Psoriasis • Dermatological disorders • Menstrual disorders Immunostimulant Anti-inflammatory Nourish blood Anti-tumor Anti-bacterial	• *S. typhi* • *E. coli* • *C. diphtheria* • *H. streptococcus*	• EtOAc fraction of *RAS* significantly inhibited NF-κB luciferase activity and TNF-α, IL-6, macrophage inflammatory protein-2 (MIP-2) and NO secretions from LPS/IFN-γ-stimulated RAW 264.7 cells.[69] • Ferulic acid from *RAS* has been shown to promote wound healing in a diabetic rat model aided by effectively inhibiting the lipid peroxidation and elevating the catalase, superoxide dismutase, glutathione, nitric oxide levels along with the increase in the serum zinc and copper levels.[70]
Jin Yin Hua (Flos Lonicerae)	• Cold • Sweet • Carbuncles • Mastitis • Pneumonia • Influenza Immunoregulation Hepatoprotective Anti-viral Anti-inflammatory Anti-bacterial	• *S. aureus* • *S. pneumoniae* • *E. coli*	• A water-soluble polysaccharide of *Flos Lonicerae* (FL) potently inhibited the picryl chloride-induced allergic contact dermatitis, leading to substantial reductions in ear thickness, serum level of IgE and histamine, as well as tissue TNF-α.[71]

(Continued)

Table 3.4.   (*Continued*)

Chinese Pin Yin Name (*Pharmaceutical Name*)	TCM Clinical Use	Pharmacological Effects	Mechanism of Action of Herbs and Active Compounds
			• Chlorogenic acid from *FL* suppresses the release of pro-inflammatory chemokine CCL7 and CXCL8 in IL-31- and IL- 33-treated eosinophils-dermal fibroblasts co-culture.[72]
Lian Qiao (*Forsythiae Fructus*)[73, 74]	• Slightly Cold • Bitter • Carbuncles • Purpura • Abscess	Antidepressant Anti-viral Anti-inflammatory Anti-bacterial • *S. aureus* • *H. pylori*	• A 70% ethanol extract of *Forsythiae Fructus* (*FF*) alleviated the AD symptoms induced by dermatophagoides farinae crude extract (DfE) in NC/Nga mouse model *in vivo*.[75] • An 80% methanol extract of *FF* (100 mg/kg) attenuated β- conglycinin-caused anaphylactic symptoms in weaned piglets *in vivo* by suppressing anaphylactic antibodies, mast cell degranulation, T lymphocyte proliferation, histamine generation, and IL-4 synthesis.[76]
Qing Dai (*Indigo Naturalis*)	• Cold • Salty • Dermatitis • Inflammatory bowel disease • Influenza • Hepatitis B	Immunoregulation Anti-inflammatory Anti-tumor Anti-bacterial • *S. aureus* • *Streptococcus*	• *Indigo Naturalis* (*IN*) differentially inhibited the proliferation of keratinocytes and endothelial cells, reduced IL-6 and IL-8, reduced the mRNA expression of anti-microbial S100A9 peptide, CCL20, chemokine, IL-1β and TNF-α cytokines in the keratinocytes treated with IL-17A. The attenuating effect of *QD* or tryptanthrin was also detected on the induced mRNA expression of several cytokines, IL-17A, IL-17F, and IL-22, during RORγT-induced TH17 polarization.[77]

			• Indigodole D, isolated from *IN*, could inhibit IL-17A protein production during the Th17 polarization or after the polarization without cytotoxicity toward Th17 cells.[78]
Zi Cao (*Radix Lithospermi*)	• Cold • Sweet • Eczema • Skin burns • Frostbite • Measles • Analgesia • Regeneration of epidermis	Anti-inflammatory Anti-viral Immunoregulation Anti-bacterial • *S. aureus* • *S. pyogenes* • *N. meningitides* • *S. typhi* • *E. coli* • *C. diphtheriae*	• *Radix Lithospermi* (*RL*) had an inhibitory effect on the atopic allergic reaction by inhibiting the release of histamine from rat peritoneal mast cells; inhibiting the anti-DNP IgE-induced passive cutaneous anaphylaxis reaction; inhibiting the increase of IL-6, IL-8, and TNF-α expression in HMC-1 cells; and inhibiting nuclear factor-kappa B (NF-κB) activation and IκB-α degradation.[79] • Deoxyshikonin from *RL* enhanced tube formation in HUVEC, and proliferation and migration in HaCaT cell by the activation of ERK and p38 MAPKs, indicating potential effectiveness in healing skin wounds for damaged tissues, such as cuts, abrasions, frostbite, and burns.[80]
Chan Tui (*Periostracum Cicadae*)	• Sweet • Cold • Dermatological disorders, including but not limited to urticaria, rash, eczema	Anti-inflammatory Vents Rashes and Relieves Itching Anti-bacterial	• The extract of *Periostracum Cicadae* (*PC*) attenuates the expression of IL-6, MMP-2, and MMP-9 in UVB-treated HaCaT cells.[81] • The administration of *PC* significantly reduces TLR4, TGF-β1, MCP-1, and IgA expression in the IgAN rats.[82]

(Continued)

Table 3.4.   (Continued)

Chinese Pin Yin Name (Pharmaceutical Name)	TCM Clinical Use	Pharmacological Effects	Mechanism of Action of Herbs and Active Compounds
			• N-acetyldopamine dimer from *Chan Tui (CT)* inhibits ROS generation, NO production, and NF-xB activity as well as the expression of pro-inflammatory molecules such as iNOS, IL-6, TNF-α, and COX-2 in LPS-induced RAW264.7 cells.[83]
Huang Bo (Cortex Phellodendri)	• Cold • Bitter • Eczema • Sores • Skin infection • Chronic bronchitis	Anti-inflammatory Anti-viral Anti-oxidant Anti-fungal Anti-bacterial • *M. bomonis* • *H. pylori*	• *Cortex Phellodendri (CP)* liniment enhanced TGF-β1, reduced MMP9 level, facilitated cell proliferation, and inhibited oxidative damage in high glucose-induced HaCaT cells, accelerating wound healing in diabetes.[84] • Berberine from *CP* could significantly suppress mast cell activation and allergic responses by inhibiting the release of β-hexosaminidase (β-HEX), histamine, IL-4 and TNF-α, and suppressing the phosphorylation of antigen-induced Lyn, Syk, and Gab2, and the MAPK pathways.[85]

mechanisms via multi-compounds and multi-targets. Recently, we conducted computational analysis on Shi Zhen Tea Ia from triple TCM therapy. Fifty-one compounds have been identified with 81 potential biological targets. We further identified the top 5 key active compounds based on molecular docking scores with hub target proteins. Besides Th1 and Th2 signaling pathways, Th17 and novel metabolic pathways such as the vitamin D receptor and peroxisome proliferator activated receptor γ (PPAR γ) are potential therapeutic targets of Shi Zhen Tea Ia against AD.[86]

In summary, TCM for treating eczema, widely used in Asia, has begun to show promising results in the US and other countries. Some studies showed safety and effectiveness in relieving itching, reducing skin inflammation, elevating quality of life, decreasing corticosteroid and antibiotic uses, and preventing recurrence. Studies have identified active compounds and elucidated underlying mechanisms. It is expected that more rigorous clinical trials, as well as further mechanistic research, will lead to FDA approval as botanical medicines.

Discussion and Conclusion

Food allergy and eczema are major public health issues and treatment options are limited. From a research perspective, TCM botanical medicines provide rich resources for advancing current therapy. Further research is needed for botanical drug development as FDA-approved standard therapies and to further define the mechanisms, following the Guidance of Industry Botanical Product from FDA (2004, updated 2016).[46] TCM herbal medicines used in practice are viewed as dietary supplements, similar to vitamins, based on the Dietary Supplement Health and Education Act of 1994 (Public Law 103-417, 103rd Congress).[47] This means that there are two parallel regulatory mechanisms. Under the supplement exception, TCM provides rich resources for integrative therapy with standard care. Although TCMs are mainly used by TCM practitioners, allergists should be able to utilize some products with high-quality control standards as well as clinical and laboratory evidence. For example, the combination of *Pruni Mume* and *Phellodendri formula* (Mei Huang Tea, 0.55g/capsule, US Times Technology Inc., Elmsford, NY) is an ethanol purified dried aqueous extract of 7 herbs that may mitigate frequent hives related to food exposure mediated by mast cell activation. *Fructus Jujubae Formula* (Digestion tea, 0.5 g/capsule, US Times Technology Inc., Elmsford, NY) is a dried aqueous extract of 6 herbs for relieving stomach pain.[28] They can also be used adjunctively for OIT or sublingual immunotherapy patients for GI symptoms. For eczema itching, skin lesions, and sleep disturbance in topical steroid dependent or steroid withdrawal patients, the triple herbal therapy described in Table 2 and our previous publication[48] may improve symptoms, quality of life, and immune responses. In addition, since these herbal remedies showed high safety profiles from clinical observational and laboratory study, together with long history of use in infants, they can be introduced as early as possible, precluding the need for topical steroid use during this period when immune systems are most vulnerable. TCM regimens for food allergy and eczema included in this review are generally well-tolerated and have high safety profiles from both clinical trials and observational studies[23-25,48] as well as laboratory studies. Lab safety test results including liver and kidney function were all in the normal range. These regimens are suitable for long-term use for chronic conditions such as food allergy and eczema in children and adults. Occasionally, they may cause stomach upset. Generally herbal medicines must be taken with food, but sometimes on an empty stomach, TCM health providers will provide detailed supervision. For children who are extremely sensitive to many things, they may have potential to react to the herbal ingredients. Thus, careful medical histories and specific protocols are needed. For chronic use, health providers should monitor clinical laboratory safety profiles every 6–12 months.

Most TCMs have anti-inflammatory actions. Added values compared with the commercially available drugs include: 1) Efficacy can be both specific and broad due to multiple compounds and targets. For example, the Forsythia formula/Shi Zhen Tea inhibits production of eotaxin, IgE, and TNF-a; 2) Most pharmaceutical drugs target specific receptors such as antihistamines, or neutralize antibodies, such as Omalizumab. TCM active compounds such as berberine directly suppressed histamine release by mast cells, and IgE production by B/plasma cells, thereby possibly changing the process of inflammation; and 3) Unlike corticosteroids, the TCM FAHF-2 and its derivatives exhibit immunomodulatory effect such as suppressing Th2, but not Th1. Therefore, TCMs may be beneficial as complementary therapy with commercial anti-allergy and anti-inflammatory drugs.

While there are substantial laboratory studies, clinical studies of food allergy and eczema are limited and sample sizes are small, so there is potential selection bias in this review. Retrospective study may have recall bias. It is also worth noting that unlike commercial drugs, TCM works slowly and therefore should not be used to treat major acute reactions by themselves. Despite these limitations, this review provides exciting evidence of TCM as integrative and complementary therapy for food allergy and steroid-dependent eczema, or dependency withdrawal. Researchers are employing advanced technologies including chromatography, systems pharmacology, and computational modeling to uncover the active compounds and molecular targets, which will ultimately lead to novel botanical medicines.

The TCM formulations and active compounds including derivatives from FAHF-2 may provide novel approaches that alter the process of food allergy by suppressing B cell IgE production and mast cell histamine release as well as TNF-α and IL-8 production. They can be used integratively with current food allergy treatment approaches such as food avoidance or OIT and SLIT to induce immune tolerance. For eczema, TCM can be used as monotherapy for infants and young children — the most vulnerable group, and may be able to spare them topical steroid treatment. Moreover, for steroid-dependent and withdrawing patients, TCM not only helps reduce infection and inflammation, but can also help skin to regain sustainable integrity. Further research is needed to address the perspectives of this study and findings.

Funding Sources

This study was supported by NIH/NCCAM Center for Complementary and Alternative Medicine grant #1R01AT001495-01A1 and 2R01 AT001495-05A2, the FA Education and Research, Winston Wolkoff Fund for Integrative Medicine for Allergies and Wellness, the Sean Parker Foundation, and General Nutraceutical Technology LLC.

Trial Registration

FAHF-2: https://ichgcp.net/clinical-trials-registry/NCT00602160
E-B-FAHF-2: https://clinicaltrials.gov/ct2/show/NCT02879006

Disclosure

Zixi Wang, Zhen-Zhen Wang, Jan Geliebter, and Raj Tiwari declare no conflicts of interest related to the current study. Xiu-Min Li received research support from the National Institutes of Health (NIH)/National Center for Complementary and Alternative Medicine (NCCAM); Food Allergy Research and Education (FARE) and Winston Wolkoff Integrative Medicine Fund for Allergies and Wellness; received consultancy fees from FARE and Johnson & Johnson Pharmaceutical Research & Development, L.L.C. Bayer HealthCare LLC; received grant from Henan University of Chinese Medicine & New York Medical College for TCM Immunopharmacology and Integrative Medicine; received royalties from UpToDate; received travel expenses from the NCCAM and FARE; received practice compensation from the Integrative Health and Acupuncture PC and US Times Technology Inc is managed by the related party; is a member of Herbs Springs, LLC, Health Freedom LLC, and General Nutraceutical Technology.

References

1. Bunyavanich S, Rifas-Shiman SL, Platts-Mills TA, *et al.* Peanut allergy prevalence among school-age children in a US cohort not selected for any disease. *J Allergy Clin Immunol.* 2014;134(3):753–755.
2. Gupta RS, Warren CM, Smith BM, *et al.* Prevalence and severity of food allergies among US adults. *JAMA Netw Open.* 2019;2(1):e185630.
3. Gupta R, Holdford D, Bilaver L, Dyer A, Holl JL, Meltzer D. The economic impact of childhood food allergy in the United States. *JAMA Pediatr.* 2013;167(11):1026–1031.
4. Moutsoglou DM, Dreskin SC. B cells establish, but do not maintain, long-lived murine anti-peanut IgE(a). *Clin Exp Allergy.* 2016;46(4):640–653.
5. Nowak-Wegrzyn A, Katz Y, Mehr SS, Koletzko S. Non-IgE-mediated gastrointestinal food allergy. *J Allergy Clin Immunol.* 2015;135(5):1114–1124.
6. Leonard SA, Pecora V, Fiocchi AG, Nowak-Wegrzyn A. Food protein-induced enterocolitis syndrome: a review of the new guidelines. *World Allergy Organ J.* 2018;11(1):4.
7. Ko J, Lee JI, Muñoz-Furlong A, Li XM, Sicherer SH. Use of complementary and alternative medicine by food-allergic patients. *Ann Allergy Asthma Immunol.* 2006;97(3):365–369.

8. Land MH, Wang J. Complementary and alternative medicine use among allergy practices: results of a nationwide survey of allergists. *J Allergy Clin Immunol Pract.* 2018;6(1):95–98.

9. Li XM. Complementary and alternative medicine for treatment of food allergy. *Immunol Allergy Clin North Am.* 2018;38(1):103–124.

10. Novak N. New insights into the mechanism and management of allergic diseases: atopic dermatitis. *Allergy.* 2009;64(2):265–275.

11. Mancini AJ, Kaulback K, Chamlin SL. The socioeconomic impact of atopic dermatitis in the United States: a systematic review. *Pediatr Dermatol.* 2008;25(1):1–6.

12. Eichenfield LF, Tom WL, Berger TG, *et al.* Guidelines of care for the management of atopic dermatitis: section 2. Management and treatment of atopic dermatitis with topical therapies. *J Am Acad Dermatol.* 2014;71(1):116–132.

13. Klonowska J, Glen J, Nowicki RJ, Trzeciak M. New cytokines in the pathogenesis of atopic dermatitisdnew therapeutic targets. *Int J Mol Sci.* 2018;19(10):3086.

14. Montes-Torres A, Llamas-Velasco M, Pérez-Plaza A, Solano-López G, SanchezPérez J. Biological treatments in atopic dermatitis. *J Clin Med.* 2015;4(4):593–613.

15. Kim HS, Yeung J. Psoriasis appearing after dupilumab therapy in atopic dermatitis: a case report. *SAGE Open Med Case Rep.* 2020;8:2050313X20940458.

16. Fahrbach K, Tarpey J, Washington EB, *et al.* Crisaborole ointment, 2%, for treatment of patients with mild-to-moderate atopic dermatitis: systematic literature review and network meta-analysis. *Dermatol Ther (Heidelb).* 2020;10(4):681–694.

17. Chen HY, Lin YH, Wu JC, *et al.* Use of traditional Chinese medicine reduces exposure to corticosteroid among atopic dermatitis children: a 1-year followup cohort study. *J Ethnopharmacol.* 2015;159:189–196.

18. Rancé F. Food allergy in children suffering from atopic eczema. *Pediatr Allergy Immunol.* 2008;19(3):279–284.

19. Langan SM, Irvine AD, Weidinger S. Atopic dermatitis. *Lancet.* 2020; 396(10247):345–360.

20. Srivastava KD, Kattan JD, Zou ZM, *et al.* The Chinese herbal medicine formula FAHF-2 completely blocks anaphylactic reactions in a murine model of peanut allergy. *J Allergy Clin Immunol.* 2005;115(1):171–178.

21. Srivastava KD, Qu C, Zhang T, Goldfarb J, Sampson HA, Li XM. Food allergy herbal formula-2 silences peanut-induced anaphylaxis for a prolonged posttreatment period via IFN-gamma-producing CD8þ T cells. *J Allergy Clin Immunol.* 2009;123(2):443–451.

22. Song Y, Qu C, Srivastava K, *et al.* Food allergy herbal formula 2 protection against peanut anaphylactic reaction is via inhibition of mast cells and basophils. *J Allergy Clin Immunol.* 2010;126(6):1208–1217.

23. Wang J, Patil SP, Yang N, *et al.* Safety, tolerability, and immunologic effects of a food allergy herbal formula in food allergic individuals: a randomized, double-blinded, placebo-controlled, dose escalation, phase 1 study. *Ann Allergy Asthma Immunol.* 2010;105(1):75–84.

24. Patil SP, Wang J, Song Y, *et al.* Clinical safety of food allergy herbal formula-2 (FAHF-2) and inhibitory effect on basophils from patients with food allergy: extended phase I study. *J Allergy Clin Immunol.* 2011;128(6):1259–1265.

25. Wang J, Jones SM, Pongracic JA, *et al.* Safety, clinical, and immunologic efficacy of a Chinese herbal medicine (food allergy herbal formula-2) for food allergy. *J Allergy Clin Immunol.* 2015;136(4):962–970.

26. Yang N, Wang J, Liu C, *et al.* Berberine and limonin suppress IgE production by human B cells and peripheral blood mononuclear cells from food-allergic patients. *Ann Allergy Asthma Immunol.* 2014;113(5):556–564.

27. Maskey A, Srivastava K, Kim M, Yang N. Analysis of biological potency and chemical consistency of ethyl acetate purified FAHF-2 for treatment of food allergy. *J Allergy Clin Immunol.* 2020;145(2):AB141.

28. Lisann L, Song Y, Wang J, Ehrlich P, Maitland A, Li XM. Successful prevention of extremely frequent and severe food anaphylaxis in three children by combined traditional Chinese medicine therapy. *Allergy Asthma Clin Immunol.* 2014;10(1):66.

29. Yamamoto T, Fujiwara K, Tsubota Y, Kageyama-Yahara N, Hayashi S, Kadowaki M. Induction of regulatory T cells as a novel mechanism underlying the therapeutic action of Kakkonto, a traditional Japanese herbal medicine, in a murine food allergy model. *Int Arch Allergy Immunol.* 2016;169(3):146–156.

30. Nagata Y, Yamamoto T, Hayashi M, Hayashi S, Kadowaki M. Improvement of therapeutic efficacy of oral immunotherapy in combination with regulatory T cell-inducer Kakkonto in a murine food allergy model. *PLoS One.* 2017;12(1):e0170577.

31. Srivastava K, Fidan O, Shi Y, *et al.* Berberine-containing natural medicine confers sustained peanut tolerance associated with distinct microbiota signature. *J Allergy Clin Immunol.* 2020;145(2):AB84.

32. Zhao G, Yang S. *Practical Diagnostic and Therapeutics and Integrated Traditional Chinese and Western Medicine.* Beijing, People's Republic of China: China Medical Science Press; 1993.

33. Thanik E, Wisniewski JA, Nowak-Wegrzyn A, Sampson H, Li XM. Effect of traditional Chinese medicine on skin lesions and quality of life in patients with moderate to severe eczema. *Ann Allergy Asthma Immunol.* 2018;121(1):135–136.

34. Yang Y, Islam MS, Wang J, Li Y, Chen X. Traditional Chinese medicine in the treatment of patients infected with 2019-new coronavirus (SARS-CoV-2): a review and perspective. *Int J Biol Sci.* 2020;16(10):1708–1717

35. Gu SX, Zhang AL, Coyle ME, Chen D, Xue CC. Chinese herbal medicine for atopic eczema: an overview of clinical evidence. *J Dermatol Treat.* 2017;28(3):246–250.

36. Srivastava K, Yang N, Uzun S, *et al.* Effect of traditional Chinese medicine (TCM) in moderate-to-severe eczema in clinic and animal model: beyond corticosteroids. *J Allergy Clin Immunol.* 2020;145(2):AB198.

37. Chen YC, Lin YH, Hu S, Chen HY. Characteristics of traditional Chinese medicine users and prescription analysis for pediatric atopic dermatitis: a population-based study. *BMC Complement Altern Med.* 2016;16:173.

38. Liu J, Mo X, Wu D, *et al.* Efficacy of a Chinese herbal medicine for the treatment of atopic dermatitis: a randomised controlled study. *Complement Ther Med.* 2015;23(5):644–651.

39. Hon KL, Leung TF, Ng PC, *et al.* Efficacy and tolerability of a Chinese herbal medicine concoction for treatment of atopic dermatitis: a randomized, double-blind, placebo-controlled study. *Br J Dermatol.* 2007;157(2):357–363.

40. Hon KL, Lo W, Cheng WK, *et al.* Prospective self-controlled trial of the efficacy and tolerability of a herbal syrup for young children with eczema. *J Dermatol Treat.* 2012;23(2):116–121.

41. Kobayashi H, Ishii M, Takeuchi S, *et al.* Efficacy and safety of a traditional herbal medicine, Hochu-ekki-to in the long-term management of Kikyo (delicate constitution) patients with atopic dermatitis: a 6-month, multicenter, doubleblind, randomized, placebo-controlled study. *Evid Based Complement Alternat Med.* 2010;7(3):367–373.

42. Ma T, Chai Y, Li S, *et al.* Efficacy and safety of Qinzhuliangxue decoction for treating atopic eczema: a randomized controlled trial. *Ann Palliat Med.* 2020;9(3):870–882.

43. Ahn JH, Yun Y, Kim MH, Ko SG, Kim KS, Choi I. Exploring the efficacy and safety of topical Jaungo application in patients with atopic dermatitis: a pilot randomized, double-blind, placebo-controlled study. *Complement Ther Med.* 2018; 40:22–28.

44. Li S, Kuchta K, Tamaru N, *et al.* Efficacy of a novel herbal multicomponent traditional Chinese medicine therapy approach in patients with atopic dermatitis. *Forsch Komplementmed.* 2013;20(3):189–196.

45. Lin PY, Chu CH, Chang FY, Huang YW, Tsai HJ, Yao TC. Trends and prescription patterns of traditional Chinese medicine use among subjects with allergic diseases: a nationwide population-based study. *World Allergy Organ J.* 2019;12(2):100001.

46. US Food and Drug Administration. Botanical drug development guidance for industry. Available at: https://www.fda.gov/downloads/Drugs/GuidanceCompliance RegulatoryInformation/Guidances/UCM458484.pdf. Accessed July 2020.

47. National Institutes of Health. Dietary Supplement Health and Education Act of 1994 Public Law 103-417d103rd Congress. Available at: https://ods.od.nih.gov/About/DSHEA_Wording.aspx. Accessed July 2020.

48. Thanik E, Wisniewski JA, Nowak-Wegrzyn A, Sampson H, Li XM. Improvement of skin lesions and life quality in moderate-to-severe eczema patients by combined TCM therapy. *Ann Allergy Asthma Immunol.* 2018;121(1):135–136.

49. Srivastava K, Yang N, Chen Y, *et al.* Efficacy, safety and immunological actions of butanol-extracted food allergy herbal formula-2 on peanut anaphylaxis. *Clin Exp Allergy.* 2011;41(4):582–591.

50. Srivastava KD, Song Y, Yang N, *et al.* B-FAHF-2 plus oral immunotherapy (OIT) is safer and more effective than OIT alone in a murine model of concurrent peanut/tree nut allergy. *Clin Exp Allergy.* 2017;47(8):1038–1049.

51. Wang Z, Kim M, Marghani Y, *et al.* Effect of E-B-FAHF-2 and 7,4'-dihydroxi-flavone (DHF) on TNF-a and IL-8 production, inflammatory markers of a nonIgE-mediated food hypersensitivity. *J Allergy Clin Immunol.* 2020;145(2):AB52.

52. Yang B, Li J, Liu X, *et al.* Herbal formula-3 inhibits food allergy in rats by stabilizing mast cells through modulating calcium mobilization. *Int Immunopharmacol.* 2013;17(3):576–584.

53. Liu S, Yang B, Yang P, Liu Z. Herbal formula-3 ameliorates OVA-induced food allergy in mice may via modulating the gut microbiota. *Am J Transl Res.* 2019;11(9):5812–5823.

54. Yamamura K, Kato S, Kato TA, *et al.* Anti-allergic mechanisms of Japanese herbal medicine, yokukansan on mast cells. *J Dermatol.* 2014;41(9):808–814.

55. Yang N, Patil S, Zhuge J, *et al.* Glycyrrhiza uralensis flavonoids present in anti-asthma formula, ASHMI, inhibit memory Th2 responses in vitro and in vivo. *Phytother Res.* 2013;27(9):1381–1391.

56. Liu C, Yang N, Chen X, *et al.* The flavonoid 7,4'-dihydroxyflavone prevents dexamethasone paradoxical adverse effect on eotaxin production by human fibroblasts. *Phytother Res.* 2017;31(3):449–458.

57. Liu C, Yang N, Song Y, *et al.* Ganoderic acid C1 isolated from the anti-asthma formula, ASHMI suppresses TNF-alpha production by mouse macrophages and peripheral blood mononuclear cells from asthma patients. *Int Immunopharmacol.* 2015;27(2):224–231.

58. Liu C, Song Y, Yang N, Tversky JR, Reid-Adam J, Li X-M. Ganoderic acid b suppressed Th2 responses and induced Th1/Tregsin cultures of peripheral blood mononuclear cells from asthmatic patients. *J Allergy Clin Immunol.* 2013;131(2):AB1.

59. Musa I, Yang N, Li X-M. Formononein isolated from Ku Shen (Radix Sophorae Flavescentis) inhibits B cell IgE production by inhibiting STAT6 and NF-kB phosphorylation and XBP1 and IgE heavy chain expression. *J Allergy Clin Immunol.* 2020;145(2):AB87.

60. Li X-M, Srivastava K, Chen Y, *et al.* Sustained silencing peanut allergy by xanthopurpurin is associated with suppression of peripheral and bone marrow IgE producing B cell. *J Allergy Clin Immunol.* 2018;141(2):AB201.

61. Cheng HM, Chiang LC, Jan YM, Chen GW, Li TC. The efficacy and safety of a Chinese herbal product (Xiao-Feng-San) for the treatment of refractory atopic dermatitis: a randomized, double-blind, placebo-controlled trial. *Int Arch Allergy Immunol.* 2011;155(2):141–148.

62. Jeong MK, Kim YE, Kim A, Jung J, Son MJ. The herbal drug, Bu-Zhong-Yi-QiTang, for the treatment of atopic dermatitis: protocol for a systematic review. *Medicine (Baltimore).* 2019;98(1):e13938.

63. Nose M, Tsutsui R, Hisaka S, *et al.* Evaluation of the safety and efficacy of Glycyrrhiza uralensis root extracts produced using artificial hydroponic and artificial hydroponic-field hybrid cultivation systems III: anti-allergic effects of hot water extracts on IgE-mediated immediate hypersensitivity in mice. *J Nat Med.* 2020;74(2):463–466.

64. Kim SH, Hong JH, Lee JE, Lee YC. 18b-Glycyrrhetinic acid, the major bioactive component of Glycyrrhizae Radix, attenuates airway inflammation by modulating Th2 cytokines, GATA-3, STAT6, and Foxp3 transcription factors in an asthmatic mouse model. *Environ Toxicol Pharmacol.* 2017;52:99–113.

65. Jayaprakasam B, Yang N, Wen MC, *et al.* Constituents of the anti-asthma herbal formula ASHMI(TM) synergistically inhibit IL-4 and IL-5 secretion by murine Th2 memory cells, and eotaxin by human lung fibroblasts in vitro. *J Integr Med.* 2013;11(3):195–205.

66. Yu M, Jia HM, Cui FX, *et al.* The effect of Chinese herbal medicine formula mKG on allergic asthma by regulating lung and plasma metabolic alternations. *Int J Mol Sci.* 2017;18(3):603.

67. Jung HS, Kim MH, Gwak NG, *et al*. Antiallergic effects of Scutellaria baicalensis on inflammation in vivo and in vitro. *J Ethnopharmacol*. 2012;141(1):345–349.

68. Shin HS, Bae MJ, Choi DW, Shon DH. Skullcap (Scutellaria baicalensis) extract and its active compound, wogonin, inhibit ovalbumin-induced Th2-mediated response. *Molecules*. 2014;19(2):2536–2545.

69. Chao WW, Hong YH, Chen ML, Lin BF. Inhibitory effects of Angelica sinensis ethyl acetate extract and major compounds on NF-kappaB trans-activation activity and LPS-induced inflammation. *J Ethnopharmacol*. 2010;129(2):244–249.

70. Ghaisas MM, Kshirsagar SB, Sahane RS. Evaluation of wound healing activity of ferulic acid in diabetic rats. *Int Wound J*. 2014;11(5):523–532.

71. Tian J, Che H, Ha D, Wei Y, Zheng S. Characterization and anti-allergic effect of a polysaccharide from the flower buds of Lonicera japonica. *Carbohydr Polym*. 2012;90(4):1642–1647.

72. Tsang MS, Jiao D, Chan BC, *et al*. Anti-inflammatory activities of pentaherbs formula, berberine, gallic acid and chlorogenic acid in atopic dermatitis-like skin inflammation. *Molecules*. 2016;21(4):519.

73. Wang Z, Xia Q, Liu X, *et al*. Phytochemistry, pharmacology, quality control and future research of Forsythia suspensa (Thunb.) Vahl: a review. *J Ethnopharmacol*. 2018;210:318–339.

74. Dong Z, Lu X, Tong X, Dong Y, Tang L, Liu M. Forsythiae Fructus: a review on its phytochemistry, quality control, pharmacology and pharmacokinetics. *Molecules*. 2017;22(9):1466.

75. Sung YY, Lee AY, Kim HK. Forsythia suspensa fruit extracts and the constituent matairesinol confer anti-allergic effects in an allergic dermatitis mouse model. *J Ethnopharmacol*. 2016;187:49–56.

76. Hao Y, Li D, Piao X, Piao X. Forsythia suspensa extract alleviates hypersensitivity induced by soybean beta-conglycinin in weaned piglets. *J Ethnopharmacol*. 2010;128(2):412–418.

77. Cheng HM, Kuo YZ, Chang CY, *et al*. The anti-TH17 polarization effect of indigo naturalis and tryptanthrin by differentially inhibiting cytokine expression. *J Ethnopharmacol*. 2020;255:112760.

78. Lee CL, Wang CM, Kuo YH, *et al*. IL-17A inhibitions of indole alkaloids from traditional Chinese medicine Qing Dai. *J Ethnopharmacol*. 2020;255:112772.

79. Kim EK, Kim EY, Moon PD, *et al*. Lithospermi radix extract inhibits histamine release and production of inflammatory cytokine in mast cells. *Biosci Biotechnol Biochem*. 2007;71(12):2886–2892.

80. Park JY, Kwak JH, Kang KS, *et al.* Wound healing effects of deoxyshikonin isolated from Jawoongo: in vitro and in vivo studies. *J Ethnopharmacol.* 2017;199:128–137.

81. Chang TM, Tsen JH, Yen H, Yang TY, Huang HC. Extract from Periostracum cicadae inhibits oxidative stress and inflammation induced by ultraviolet B irradiation on HaCaT keratinocytes. *Evid Based Complement Alternat Med.* 2017;2017:8325049.

82. Yang L, Wang Y, Nuerbiye A, *et al.* Effects of periostracum cicadae on cytokines and apoptosis regulatory proteins in an IgA nephropathy rat model. *Int J Mol Sci.* 2018;19(6):1599.

83. Xu MZ, Lee WS, Han JM, *et al.* Antioxidant and anti-inflammatory activities of N-acetyldopamine dimers from Periostracum Cicadae. *Bioorg Med Chem.* 2006;14(23):7826–7834.

84. Zhang J, Zhou R, Xiang C, Jia Q, Wu H, Yang H. Huangbai liniment accelerated wound healing by activating Nrf2 signaling in diabetes. *Oxid Med Cell Longev.* 2020;2020:4951820.

85. Fu S, Ni S, Wang D, Fu M, Hong T. Berberine suppresses mast cell-mediated allergic responses via regulating FceRI-mediated and MAPK signaling. *Int Immunopharmacol.* 2019;71:1–6.

86. Wang ZZ, Jia Y, Srivastava KD, Huang W, Tiwari R, Nowak-Wegrzyn A, Geliebter J, Miao M, Li XM. Systems pharmacology and in silico docking analysis uncover association of CA2, PPARG, RXRA, and VDR with the mechanisms underlying the Shi Zhen Tea formula effect on eczema. *Evid Based Complement Alternat Med.* 2021 May 13; 2021: 8406127. DOI: 10.1155/2021/8406127

87. Kattan JD, Srivastava KD, Zou MZ. Pharmacological and immunological effects of individual herbs in the Food Allergy Herbal Formula-2 (FAHF-2) on peanut allergy. *Phytother Res.* 2008;22(5):651–659.

BRIEF OUTLINE OF CHINESE MEDICINE'S UNDERSTANDING AND TREATMENT OF DERMATOLOGICAL DISEASE

Mazin Al-Khafaji*

Doctor of Chinese Medicine, Shanghai, China

Chinese medicine (CM) has a long, rich, and distinguished history reaching back into antiquity, not only in treating but also categorizing the widest range of skin disease. There is no other area of specialty within CM that comes so close to modern biomedicine as the classification and diagnosis of dermatological disorders. This is easy to understand given that both systems have, to a very great degree, relied upon on close study of the presentation and morphology in cataloging skin disease, so much so that by the late 17th century some 360 disease entities were recognized that very closely mirror

---

* Mazin Al-Khafaji is a TCM practitioner at the Avicenna Center for Chinese Medicine, UK. He is a master herbalist and recognized as one of the leading clinicians and teachers in the field of dermatology and Chinese medicine. Over the past three decades he has taught his successful and innovative approach to clinical practice to thousands of students worldwide.

modern-day classification. Certainly, conditions such as psoriasis, lichen planus, pompholyx eczema, impetigo, herpes zoster and so on, were well described, but also rare autoimmune conditions such as the blistering family of disease of pemphigus and pemphigoid. Conditions such as scleroderma and morphea were named, and treatment protocols advanced. There was even a clear reference to what must have been a rare condition in the pre-industrial era — 450 years ago — when the name "wind of the four crooks" (四灣風) was first coined to describe what today we call eczema.

Although CM has relied on a different paradigm to understand the natural process in the world around us, it is, nonetheless, a highly scientific model in the true sense of the word. Over several millennia it has amassed an enormous amount of clinically relevant and nuanced insights, constructed into rational, internally consistent and coherent concepts that underpin understanding of how a healthy body-mind functions and what happens when disease arises, and crucially how to approach, via reasoned and methodical protocols, sound methods to restore health.

To the uninitiated, the theories that have evolved in CM to construct a diagnosis, understand the pathology of disease, and determine protocols for their treatment are often dismissed as being arcane and of no value in the modern day of advanced reductionist science.

In fact, these abstractions are highly refined and subtle concepts that ultimately inform the doctor how to combine a whole range of disparate ingredients (a typical CM dispensary will have 500+ ingredients) — each ingredient containing a multitude of active compounds — to permit construction of an efficacious formula of herbs. Typically, 12–15 ingredients are cooked into a decoction. Together, the synergetic action of the multiple active constituents combats the disease state and restores the body-mind system to a stable equilibrium that we call health.

I believe that to dismiss these evolved concepts as antiquated and worthless is a significant mistake. Seemingly simplistic concepts have evolved from layered human experience, reflecting very insightful observations acquired over millennia. The clinically relevant accumulated knowledge and insights are a treasure house of expertise not easy to acquire other than through practical experience over extended periods of time. This is especially the case when attempting to fathom the vastly complex interaction of disparate plant substances and their multifarious active compounds that belie their potency, often only revealing their potential when multiple ingredients are combined into a formula.

There is very little space here to do anything but allude to the contrasting paradigm of CM and its elaborate and refined theoretical framework, but I would like to highlight just two elements.

First, clearly an ancient people would very reasonably have borrowed concepts from nature all around them to describe the clinical events they perceived. So, metaphors evolved to act as a distinct and nuanced language, not only in describing the complexities of the presenting disease, but crucially to begin the elaborate process of constructing the all-important formula of ingredients to suit that particular pattern of presentation. These include *heat* (very similar to a dry non-exudative inflammatory processes); *dampness* (roughly oedematose inflammation with exudate, as well as when the pathological changes primarily affect the lower body or intertriginous areas); *wind* (corresponding to certain forms of pruritis, epidermal as opposed to dermal changes, as well as when the pathological changes primarily affect the upper body); *dryness* (malnourished dry, fissured skin as, for example so often seen in eczema); *toxin* (includes bacterial or viral infections). The Materia medica of primarily plant and mineral ingredients are also designated actions that counter these pathological entities (so, for example, there are multiple ingredients that clear *heat*, in other words reduce dry inflammation; scatter *wind*, alleviating itch; resolve *toxin*, to possess anti-bacterial or anti-viral properties and so on).

Secondly, and of an even higher priority, the understanding of disease in a broader context, where the emphasis is not just in controlling the more acute manifestations, but the pivotal aim of restoring a stable equilibrium to a diseased state once the treatment is withdrawn. In fact, this above all else most starkly defines the different approaches between modern biomedicine and CM.

If we take as an example a typical chronic inflammatory disease such as eczema or psoriasis to illustrate this, we can say whereas the emphasis in modern medicine is at reducing and eliminating the inflammatory process by a range of methods commensurate with the severity of the disease, so anything from simple emollients as the lowest rung, through topical steroids or tacrolimus, to internal steroids, immunosuppressives or the biologics (so too the pharmaceuticals that target the primary pathways that are engaged at the onset of inflammation). All but the first of these can be thought of as a palliative approach, where in essence the inflammatory pathways are identified to a greater or lesser degree and then blocked. Whereas this may be a successful approach in the short term, in more entrenched conditions, once the medicine is withdrawn, the body's previous status quo quickly reinstates itself and inflammation runs rampant once again.

In CM on the other hand, the acute manifestations of these chronic inflammatory diseases are recognized as one of three states the body can occupy. The first stage in treatment, known as the draining phase, will involve controlling the persistent active inflammation (so from CM perspective such methods as clearing *heat*, drying *dampness*, scattering *wind*, resolving *toxin* and so on are employed, depending on the specific manifestation in an individual patient — so truly an individualized approach must be applied to achieve results), but that would be considered the first port of call.

Once that is achieved and much of the inflammation controlled, what ensues is in fact the most involved, refined and distinctive phase of treatment, namely, to reestablish a stable homoeostasis, by in effect segueing from the draining phase, in increments, through what in CM is referred to as the harmonizing phase (which amounts to a mixture of subduing the inflammation and beginning the all-important restoring of the aberrant immune function to normal).

Once that is achieved, the final and third stage of treatment, the tonifying phase, is initiated. In this phase, the restored, correctly functioning immune system is secured in its healthy state by yet a different formulation.

This three-phase application is crucial for success, so, for example, if the tonification phase is applied prematurely at the outset when inflammation is pronounced, no benefit will be achieved; indeed, the inflammatory process will almost certainly be activated.

I would venture that the secondary and tertiary phases of treatment in Chinese medicine, whose functions are to secure the elusive stable state where persistent inflammation is cleared, has more in common with the mechanisms and pathways that have more recently been identified in modern medicine — the active processes, regulated by biochemical mediators and receptor signaling pathways driven by specialized pro-resolving mediators (SPMs) such as *Resolvins*, *Protectins*, *Lipoxins* etc. — rather than in the initial phases of subduing inflammation.

In summary, the following three phases act as a template to follow in escorting diseased states from the persistent inflammatory phases to resolution and stability.

Phase I (Draining Method) — Subdue inflammation.

Phase II (Harmonizing Method) — Restore aberrant system to a stable state, and at the same time ensure that the inflammation continues to be held in check.

Phase III (Tonifying Method) — Consolidate the changes, often no or only a few ingredients to control active inflammation are used (as by this phase they are no longer needed) so that on withdrawing the medicine, equilibrium is maintained.

So, to summarize, Chinese medicine's approach in tackling inflammatory conditions of the skin (in fact this applies to pretty much all inflammatory disease, such as ulcerative colitis, rheumatoid arthritis) is not a single approach, using a single formula of herbs. Rather it's a dynamic process which utilizes a whole range of appropriate ingredients, chosen by an elaborate and intricate theoretical framework that links the specifics of the pathological manifestation of the diseased process with clinically tried and tested combination of ingredients that will resolve them. This is achieved by regularly altering the formula of ingredients at the appropriate time to guide the ecology of the body-mind system from a diseased state to a healthy one, thus maximizing the chance of this stability to endure once the treatment is withdrawn.

MECHANISM OF ECZEMA, BIOMARKERS, AND PERSPECTIVES OF TCM THERAPEUTIC TARGETS

Kamal D. Srivastava, PhD and Xiu-Min Li, MD, MS

Department of Pathology, Microbiology and Immunology,
and Department of Otolaryngology
New York Medical College, Valhalla, New York 10595, USA

Abstract

Atopic dermatitis, commonly referred to as eczema, is a heterogenous skin condition marked by chronic severe itchy and inflamed skin. Recent developments in the fields of genetics, microbiome research, and molecular diagnostics have elucidated complex interactions between skin, the immune system, and skin microbiome that drive eczema. In this chapter, we review current understanding of eczema mechanisms, biomarkers and discuss recent studies highlighting modern analytical and in silico modeling approaches that shed new light on therapeutic targets of active compounds present in TCM eczema formulas.

Keywords: Atopic dermatitis, eczema, microbiome, biomarkers, in silico modeling.

Current Understanding of Eczema Mechanisms

Eczema is a chronic inflammatory skin condition that is often non-responsive to standard treatment such as steroids.[1] We now appreciate that the mechanisms driving its pathophysiology are more than skin-deep. A complex interplay between dysfunctional skin barrier, skin microbiome disturbances, and predominantly type-2-skewed immune dysregulation works in a multidirectional way to bring about hallmark eczema symptoms such as itching, redness, oozing lesions, and dermal thickening.[1] A suboptimal skin barrier leads to epidermal water loss and aberrant colonization by pathogenic bacteria, promoting inflammation and Tcell infiltration.[2] Colonization with pathogens such as *Staphylococcus aureus* damages the skin barrier and induces innate inflammatory responses and local Th2 immune responses.[3] Th2-skewed systemic immune responses influence the skin microbiome and cutaneous inflammatory cells such as mast cells.[3] Thus, the skin, microbiome, and systemic immune responses form 3 key mechanistic pillars of eczema.

Skin Defects in Eczema

A major function of skin is to provide an effective barrier against harmful external exposures.[4] It serves to limit passive water loss, while protecting against environmental and chemical exposures. Compromised skin barrier is a foundational mechanism in eczema. Skin lipids such as ceramides and proteins relevant to epidermal differentiation such as filaggrin, loricrin, and corneodesmosin are frequently altered in eczema patients, even in non-lesional skin.[5,6] Itchy skin is a major eczema symptom. Local skin immune responses in eczema include infiltration of Th2 cells, eosinophils, neutrophils, and activation of cutaneous mast cells. These release pro-inflammatory cytokines and peptides that activate itch receptors on sensory neurons present in abundance in the skin. One of the best-known mediators of pruritus is IL-31 which is produced by Th2 cells.[7,8] Classical Th2 cytokines IL-4 and IL-13 have also been reported to contribute to the itch-scratch cycle as evidenced by presence of receptors for IL-4 and IL-13 on sensory neurons.[9]

Systemic Immune Responses in Eczema

For eczema that can be characterized as atopic dermatitis, a pro-Th2 skewed systemic immune response is a major disease driver.[3,9] Pro-Th2 mediators and cytokines include TSLP, IL-33, IL-4, IL-5, and IL-13.[10] Th2-skewed immune system is instrumental to establishing the allergic immune milieu and setting the stage for development of eczema. IL-4 and IL-13 cause reduced antimicrobial peptide production by skin cells, which is thought to promote colonization by pathogenic bacteria such as *Staphylococcus aureus*. Once the disease enters the chronic phase, Th1 and Th2 cytokines participate in cutaneous inflammation and epidermal thickening respectively.[3] That non-lesional skin in eczema patients also displays aberrant cytokine profile points to the systemic nature of immune dysregulation in eczema. A study by the Guttman-Yassky group showed that early onset eczema in young children showed Th17 and Th9 polarization in addition to Th2-skewed responses.[11]

The Microbiome in Eczema

Healthy skin supports a diverse array of commensal bacteria and other microbes.[12,13] Eczematous skin, especially during flares, shows decreased microbial diversity and reduced production of antimicrobial peptides.[1] A majority of eczema patients show skin colonization with pathogenic *Staphylococcus aureus* which is now considered an eczema biomarker. *S. aureus* has been shown to stimulate production of key eczema drivers such as TSLP and other Th2 cytokines.[3,14,15] Factors that promote overgrowth of *S. aureus* are still being understood but disturbances in skin integrity and decreased production of cutaneous antimicrobial peptides have been implicated.[15,16] The fungus Malassezia has been shown to colonize eczematous skin, especially in eczema of the head and neck. Harmful microbes activate innate inflammatory pathways raising the level of several cytokines such as IL-beta and TNF-a, which play a role in eczema flares. Additionally, eczema patients frequently mount IgE responses to microbial antigens such as the case with *S. aureus* and Malassezia.[16]

Eczema Biomarkers

Biomarkers are measurable substances in the body or quantifiable observations that inform about the presence or progression of a disease.[17,18] Biomarkers can provide useful information for disease diagnosis, prognosis, and prediction or monitoring of treatment responses.[18] Biomarker based disease stratification identifies clinically relevant subgroups and aids development of targeted therapies. Efficient biomarker identification has proven to be a major catalyst for treatment advances for diseases like asthma and cancer.[19] We are at the doorstep of a similar revolution for eczema. The past few years have witnessed a concerted effort to discover and validate useful eczema biomarkers,[20,21] allowing clinicians to better understand eczema types and tailor personalized treatment approaches, thus offering treatment beyond standard eczema care that largely relies topical and systemic steroids. Key, mechanistically important eczema biomarkers are discussed below.

Systemic Immune Biomarkers

Determination and validation of serum biomarkers in eczema has led to identification of several biomarkers that have increased our appreciation for the heterogenous nature of the disease as well as provided valuable therapeutic targets. The classical Th2 cytokines IL-4 and IL-13 are accepted biomarkers for a large portion of eczema patients and are targeted by the biologic dupilumab.[17,22] Bakker *et al.* used serum biomarkers to reveal 4 distinct eczema clusters, namely "skin-homing chemokines/IL-1R1-dominant" cluster, "TH1/TH2/TH17-dominant" cluster, "TH2/TH22/PARC-dominant" cluster, and a "TH2/eosinophil-inferior" cluster.[18]

Skin Biomarkers

Physical and structural properties of skin have been used as clinical biomarkers for eczema. Transepidermal Water Loss (TEWL) measured from skin is a robust eczema biomarker.[23,24] Higher rates of water loss from skin are highly correlated with eczema severity.[25] Epidermal thickness, assessed by histological examination of skin biopsy is also an informative eczema biomarker. However, associated pain and issues with post-biopsy healing have spurred development of tape-stripping methods to obtain gene expression data.[26,27] Using this method, skin expression of Th2 cytokines, filaggrin, Th22 and IL17 among others were validated as skin biomarkers of eczema.[26]

Microbial Biomarkers

Overall, microbial diversity is reduced in eczematous skin.[9] Over 90% of eczema patients show overgrowth of *S. aureus* in lesional skin suggesting that presence of *S. aureus* is a robust microbial biomarker for eczema.[3] This is a mechanistically important biomarker as well, since *S. aureus* perpetuates Th2 responses by stimulating production of TSLP, IL-4 and IL-13.[3] The fungus Malassezia has also been implicated in eczema, especially in eczema involving head and neck regions. Specific IgE responses to *S. aureus* and Malassezia antigens are common in eczema patients.[15,24]

TCM and Eczema Therapeutic Targets

Eczema and other skin disorders have been recognized in TCM for several centuries.[28] As TCM becomes more widely accepted throughout the world, modern approaches to understanding mechanisms and molecular targets are advancing our understanding of how these multi-herb formulas work.[29] In a review by Wang *et al.*,[30] top 10 TCM herbs, such as Angelica sinensis, Sophora flavesence and Glycyrrhiza uralensis, found in TCM eczema formulas were discussed and immunomodulatory and anti-pruritic actions of these herbs were highlighted. In another study, the eczema formula, Shi Zhen Tea (SZT) developed by Dr. Xiu-Min Li — inspired by Xiao Feng San, an acclaimed TCM formula in China documented in *Orthodox Manual of External Medicine* — eliminates itching in the body. The Li research group reported excellent efficacy of SZT in treatment of eczema.[31] Using systems pharmacology based on network analysis, molecular mechanisms of SZT were predicted using herb feature mapping, drug target mining, network and pathway analyses, and in silico molecular docking.[32] The group found that SZT efficacy in eczema could be attributed to immune and metabolic functions via regulation of multiple pathways and networks. Among these, four key pathways stood out, including Th17 cell differentiation, pathways in cancer, metabolic pathways, and PI3K-Akt signaling pathway. Molecular docking studies between active compounds and proteins CA2, PPARG, RXRA, and Vitamin D Receptor confirmed moderate to strong binding affinities.[32]

Conclusions and Future Perspectives

Recognition of eczema as a heterogenous complex disease has allowed for broadening of knowledge related to underlying mechanisms that drive the disease which is paving the way for development of more targeted treatments that are urgently needed as standard care (steroids) often fails many eczema patients. Ongoing research of eczema mechanisms and biomarkers suggests that a multi-pronged approach may be needed as multiple systems of the body such as skin, immune system, and microbiome interact to bring about eczema symptoms. TCM and its multi-herb formulas are ideally positioned to provide a comprehensive multi-targeted approach to eczema treatment, especially for those who do not benefit from standard steroid therapy. Modern analytical and in silico modeling approaches are now shedding light on potential targets of active compounds present in efficacious formulas such as SZT. Future clinical trials of simplified formulas or compound enriched fractions may allow for wide acceptance of these traditional formulas in Western countries.

References

1. Langan SM, Irvine AD, Weidinger S. Atopic dermatitis. *Lancet.* Aug 1 2020;396(10247):345–360. doi:10.1016/s0140-6736(20)31286-1
2. Fleischer DM, Udkoff J, Borok J, *et al.* Atopic dermatitis: Skin care and topical therapies. *Semin Cutan Med Surg.* Sep 2017;36(3):104–110. doi:10.12788/j. sder.2017.035
3. Guttman-Yassky E, Krueger JG, Lebwohl MG. Systemic immune mechanisms in atopic dermatitis and psoriasis with implications for treatment. *Exp Dermatol.* Apr 2018;27(4):409–417. doi: 10.1111/exd.13336
4. Yang G, Seok JK, Kang HC, Cho YY, Lee HS, Lee JY. Skin barrier abnormalities and immune dysfunction in atopic dermatitis. *Int J Mol Sci.* Apr 20 2020;21(8)doi: 10.3390/ijms21082867

5. Bhattacharya N, Sato WJ, Kelly A, Ganguli-Indra G, Indra AK. Epidermal lipids: Key mediators of atopic dermatitis pathogenesis. *Trends Mol Med.* Jun 2019;25(6):551–562. doi: 10.1016/j.molmed.2019.04.001

6. Simpson ELMM, Irvine ADM, Eichenfield LFM, Friedlander SFM. Update on epidemiology, diagnosis, and disease course of atopic dermatitis. *Semin Cutan Med Surg.* Jun 2016;35(5 Suppl):S84–88. doi: 10.12788/j.sder.2016.041

7. Lee CH, Yu HS. Biomarkers for itch and disease severity in atopic dermatitis. *Curr Probl Dermatol.* 2011;41:136–148. doi: 10.1159/000323307

8. Moyle M, Cevikbas F, Harden JL, Guttman-Yassky E. Understanding the immune landscape in atopic dermatitis: The era of biologics and emerging therapeutic approaches. *Exp Dermatol.* Jul 2019;28(7):756–768. doi: 10.1111/exd.13911

9. Sroka-Tomaszewska J, Trzeciak M. Molecular mechanisms of atopic dermatitis pathogenesis. *Int J Mol Sci.* Apr 16 2021;22(8)doi: 10.3390/ijms22084130

10. Sugita K, Akdis CA. Recent developments and advances in atopic dermatitis and food allergy. *Allergol Int.* Apr 2020;69(2):204–214. doi: 10.1016/j. alit.2019.08.013

11. Esaki H, Brunner PM, Renert-Yuval Y, *et al.* Early-onset pediatric atopic dermatitis is T(H)2 but also T(H)17 polarized in skin. *J Allergy Clin Immunol.* Dec 2016;138(6):1639–1651. doi: 10.1016/j.jaci.2016.07.013

12. Pascal M, Perez-Gordo M, Caballero T, *et al.* Microbiome and allergic diseases. *Front Immunol.* 2018;9:1584. doi:10.3389/fimmu.2018.01584

13. Wesemann DR, Nagler CR. The microbiome, timing, and barrier function in the context of allergic disease. *Immunity.* Apr 19 2016;44(4):728–738. doi: 10.1016/j.immuni.2016.02.002

14. Reiger M, Traidl-Hoffmann C, Neumann AU. The skin microbiome as a clinical biomarker in atopic eczema: Promises, navigation, and pitfalls. *J Allergy Clin Immunol.* Jan 2020;145(1):93–96. doi: 10.1016/j.jaci.2019.11.004

15. Bjerre RD, Bandier J, Skov L, Engstrand L, Johansen JD. The role of the skin microbiome in atopic dermatitis: a systematic review. *Br J Dermatol.* Nov 2017;177(5):1272–1278. doi: 10.1111/bjd.15390

16. Mittermann I, Wikberg G, Johansson C, *et al.* IgE Sensitization profiles differ between adult patients with severe and moderate atopic dermatitis. *PLoS One.* 2016;11(5):e0156077. doi: 10.1371/journal.pone.0156077

17. Renert-Yuval Y, Thyssen JP, Bissonnette R, *et al.* Biomarkers in atopic dermatitis-a review on behalf of the International Eczema Council. *J Allergy Clin Immunol.* Jan 28 2021;doi: 10.1016/j.jaci.2021.01.013

18. Bakker DS, Nierkens S, Knol EF, *et al.* Confirmation of multiple endotypes in atopic dermatitis based on serum biomarkers. *J Allergy Clin Immunol.* Jan 2021;147(1):189–198. doi: 10.1016/j.jaci.2020.04.062

19. Silkoff PE, Strambu I, Laviolette M, *et al*. Asthma characteristics and biomarkers from the Airways Disease Endotyping for Personalized Therapeutics (ADEPT) longitudinal profiling study. *Respir Res.* Nov 17 2015;16:142. doi: 10.1186/s12931-015-0299-y

20. Mohapatra SS, Mohapatra S, McGill AR, Green R. Molecular mechanism-driven new biomarkers and therapies for atopic dermatitis. *J Allergy Clin Immunol.* Jul 2020;146(1):72–73. doi: 10.1016/j.jaci.2020.04.039

21. Thijs JL, de Bruin-Weller MS, Hijnen D. Current and future biomarkers in atopic dermatitis. *Immunol Allergy Clin North Am.* Feb 2017;37(1):51–61. doi: 10.1016/j.iac.2016.08.008

22. Nakahara T, Izuhara K, Onozuka D, *et al*. Exploration of biomarkers to predict clinical improvement of atopic dermatitis in patients treated with dupilumab: A study protocol. *Medicine (Baltimore).* Sep 18 2020;99(38):e22043. doi: 10.1097/md.0000000000022043

23. Brunner PM, Israel A, Leonard A, *et al*. Distinct transcriptomic profiles of early-onset atopic dermatitis in blood and skin of pediatric patients. *Ann Allergy Asthma Immunol.* Mar 2019;122(3):318–330.e3. doi: 10.1016/j.anai.2018.11.025

24. Hon KL, Tsang KY, Kung JS, Leung TF, Lam CW, Wong CK. Clinical signs, Staphylococcus and atopic eczema-related seromarkers. *Molecules.* Feb 14 2017;22(2)doi: 10.3390/molecules22020291

25. Flohr C, England K, Radulovic S, *et al*. Filaggrin loss-of-function mutations are associated with early-onset eczema, eczema severity and transepidermal water loss at 3 months of age. *Br J Dermatol.* Dec 2010;163(6):1333–1336.

26. Dyjack N, Goleva E, Rios C, *et al*. Minimally invasive skin tape strip RNA sequencing identifies novel characteristics of the type 2-high atopic dermatitis disease endotype. *J Allergy Clin Immunol.* Apr 2018;141(4):1298–1309. doi: 10.1016/j.jaci.2017.10.046

27. Amarbayasgalan T, Takahashi H, Dekio I, Morita E. Interleukin-8 content in the stratum corneum as an indicator of the severity of inflammation in the lesions of atopic dermatitis. *Int Arch Allergy Immunol.* 2013;160(1):63–74. doi: 10.1159/000339666

28. Wang Z, Wang ZZ, Geliebter J, *et al*. Traditional Chinese medicine for food allergy and eczema. *Ann Allergy Asthma Immunol.* 2021 Jun;126(6):639-654.

29. Srivastava K, Yang N, Uzun S, *et al*. Effect of traditional Chinese medicine (TCM) in moderate-to-severe eczema in clinic and animal model: beyond corticosteroids. *The Journal of Allergy and Clinical Immunology.* 2020;145(2):AB198.

30. Wang Z, Wang ZZ, Geliebter J, *et al*. Traditional Chinese medicine for food allergy and eczema. *Ann Allergy Asthma Immunol.* 2021 Jun;126(6):639-654.

31. Uzun S, Wang Z, McKnight TA, *et al.* Improvement of skin lesions in corticosteroid withdrawal-associated severe eczema by multicomponent traditional Chinese medicine therapy. *Allergy, Asthma & Clinical Immunology.* 2021;Accepted

32. Wang ZZ, Jia Y, Srivastava KD, *et al.* Systems pharmacology and in silico docking analysis uncover association of CA2, PPARG, RXRA, and VDR with the mechanisms underlying the Shi Zhen Tea formula effect on eczema. *Evid Based Complement Alternat Med.* 2021;2021:8406127. doi: 10.1155/2021/8406127

THE ROLE OF MICROBIOTA IN ECZEMA

Jan Geliebter, PhD*, Xiu-Min Li, MD, MS, and Raj Tiwari, PhD*

*Department of Pathology, Microbiology and Immunology,
and Department of Otolaryngology
New York Medical College, Valhalla, New York 10595, USA*

Introduction

Eczema is a disease characterized by defects in skin integrity, immune dysregulation and alterations in the microbiota, including colonization/infection with *Staphylococcus aureus* on the skin.[1-3] Thus, this disease involves multiple interacting components, making the identification of the key, initiating, targetable component difficult. For example, the overproduction of IL-4 down-regulates the production of key skin integrity components, including filaggrin, as well as decreasing antibacterial peptide production by these cells.[1-5] This allows for the entry of allergens and bacteria, such as *S. aureus*, exacerbating the disease. *S. aureus* has been shown to down-regulate the production of antibacterial peptides, facilitating colonization and subsequent pathologic events, furthering both reductions in skin integrity and the dysregulated Th2 immune response. Predisposing genetic mutations, such as in the filaggrin gene itself, have been shown to permit increased skin permeability, also facilitating the entry of allergens, and changing the environment and constituents

---

* Professor

of the skin microbiota. Thus, eczema represents a vicious cycle of interacting immunological and microbiological factors, which are visible on the skin, but also have systemic implications, including cardiovascular disease.[1,6]

Microbiota and Immune System

The interactions between our normal, commensal microorganisms and our immune system are fascinating, and still represent an under-explored and inadequately understood frontier. Further, microbiota at distinct anatomical sites do not work in isolation from one other, affecting each other and our local and systemic immune responses, as well as affecting many physiologic systems and disease states.[7]

The maternal gut microbiota and their bacterial metabolic products are key to the normal development of the fetal immune system.[8–11] The maternal microbiome prepares the fetal immune system for entry into a world filled with microorganisms. Specifically, the developing immune system of the fetus must be prepared to act and react when, shortly after birth, it is rapidly colonized by microorganisms that can wreak havoc on a naïve or dysregulated immune environment. A balance between overreaction (inflammation, allergy, eczema, autoimmunity) and tolerance (to self, foreign — but not dangerous material such as food) must be initiated before birth and carefully developed and maintained afterwards. Much of the immunomodulatory effect of gut microbiota is effected through the induction of Treg cells that promote an immunosuppressive environment on the mucosal surfaces.[8,11]

Skin Microbiota and Skin Integrity

As prefaced above, the dysregulated immune response and skin integrity of eczema are greatly modulated by the microbiota. However, we are only beginning to understand the relationship between microbiota and eczema. Of interest are the microbiota of the gut, skin and other systems, and the absolute and relative bacterial, fungal and viral components.

As reviewed by Thomas and Fernadez-Penas[4] and Kim and Kim,[7] normal skin exhibits significant microbiological diversity, and varies with an individual's age and body site. At the phylum level, the skin contains predominantly Actinobacteria, Firmicutes, Proteobacteria and Bacteroides, and at the genus level Cutibacteria (Propionibacteria), Streptococcus, Staphylococcus aureus (S. aureus), Corynebacterium and Lactobacillus. Additionally, microbiota differ on the skin location with Cutibacterium found at sebaceous sites and Staphylococcus and Corynebacterium localizing to moist areas.[7,12] Significantly, lesional sites exhibit decreased amounts of "protective" bacteria such as Cutibacteria, Corynebacterium and others.[7,13,14] In addition, filaggrin defects have been demonstrated to provide a more favorable environment for *S. aureus* binding and colonization by inducing alterations in corneocytes that facilitate their binding.

The diversity of the microbiota at the species level is significant as *S. aureus* and *S. epidermitis* are believed to have opposing effects in normal skin, as well as in eczema.[4,7,15] For example, *S. epidermitis* produces antimicrobial peptides that inhibit the growth of *S. aureus* and other pathogens, while *S. aureus* inhibits production of antimicrobial compounds by epithelial cells. *S. epidermitis* also inhibits the growth of *S. aureus* by the production of porphyrin.[4,7] However, *S. epidermitis* has been positively associated with SCORAD, so the roles and relationships of various bacterial species represent a complex issue.[16]

S. aureus carriage has been reported in up to 100% in eczema patients compared to ~20 in normal controls.[7,17] Further, *S. aureus* has been reported to be increased in lesional vs. non-lesional skin and decreases upon treatment.[4,7] Taking taxonomy to an even deeper level, different strains of *S. aureus* have been reported to be carried by eczema patients compared to control populations.[7,14] *S. aureus* may also contribute to itching as it induces apoptosis in keratinocytes, resulting in the release of thymic stromal lymphopoietin and further skews the aberrant Th2 immune response.[7,18]

Gut Microbiota

Microbial diversity in the gut is associated with a healthier phenotype. Numerous studies of the gut microbiota have suggested that lower levels of Bifidobacteria, Akkermansia and Faecalibacterium and higher levels of *E. coli*, Clostridia and Staphylococcus are associated with eczema and even more pronounced during flares.[4,7,19–21] Similar to the skin, the gut microbiota begins to be formed at delivery and progressively changes during the first few years of life. The diversity and composition at each stage will depend on variables such as vaginal vs. caesarean section, breast vs. formula fed and the introduction to solid food.[7] As reviewed by Kim and Kim[7] vaginal birth is associated with beneficial commensals, including species of Bacteroides and Bifidbacterium, while caesarean birth is associated with Streptococcus, Staphylococcus and *C. difficile*. In a similar manner, breast-feeding is associated with Bifidobacteria colonization, while *E. coli* and Clostridium are associated with bottle-feeding.[7]

Beneficial or "normalized" gut microbiota includes species that are associated with decreased inflammation, to a large extent working through bacterial metabolites such as short chain fatty acids that modulate the development of a more regulated, less inflammatory, immune system. This is accomplished by several mechanisms, primarily through the skewing of T cell development towards the Treg, immunosuppressive phenotype.[7,22,23] Treg cells prevent the maturation of other T cells, decrease eosinophil and mast cell activity and IgE production.[7]

Probiotic Therapy

While data concerning the relationship between eczema and microbiota are accumulating, our current understanding is insufficient to utilize microbial therapy for the treatment of eczema. Results on the use of various "beneficial" bacterial interventions such as probiotics has yielded inconclusive and conflicting results.[7] Most significantly, meta-analysis of reports has failed to show beneficial effects of probiotics on symptoms of eczema.[24] These results may be due to many factors.[7] For example, the lack of taxonomic analysis down to the species and strain level is critical. In addition to *S. aureus* vs. *S. epidermitis* mentioned above, different strains of *S. aureus* have been observed in flare skin sites vs. non-flare. Different species of Bifidobacteria have been positively and negatively associated with eczema.

Future Prospects

Some key caveats of past and current studies, as well as guidance for future research, have been presented by Reiger *et al.*[26] For example, are relative frequencies of bacteria (at any taxonomic level) sufficient for analysis or are absolute microbial loads necessary? If absolute amounts are required, what should be the "standardized" skin area analyzed? What should be the standard for skin sampling? Is 16S NGS sampling sufficient or do we need more quantitative methods such as qPCR? As discussed above, deeper taxonomic investigation may be necessary. Also, to what extent do the fungal and viral microbiota play a role in skin (and systemic) health and dysfunction? As more "standardized" information is obtained, or more importantly, analyzed, significant breakthroughs in the role of the microbiota in eczema at all stages of life will be made, along with microbial therapy of the disease.

References

1. Brunner PM, Guttman-Yassky E, Leung DY. The immunology of atopic dermatitis and its reversibility with broad-spectrum and targeted therapies. *J Allergy Clin Immunol*. 2017 Apr;139(4S):S65–S76. doi: 10.1016/j.jaci.2017.01.011. PMID: 28390479
2. Czarnowicki T, He H, Krueger JG, Guttman-Yassky E. Atopic dermatitis endotypes and implications for targeted therapeutics. *J Allergy Clin Immunol*. 2019 Jan;143(1):1–11. doi: 10.1016/j.jaci.2018.10.032. PMID: 30612663
3. Peng W, Novak N. Pathogenesis of atopic dermatitis. *Clin Exp Allergy*. 2015 Mar;45(3):566–574. doi: 10.1111/cea.12495. PMID: 25610977
4. Thomas CL, Fernández-Peñas P. The microbiome and atopic eczema: More than skin deep. *Australas J Dermatol*. 2017 Feb;58(1):18–24. doi: 10.1111/ajd.12435. Epub 2016 Jan 28. PMID: 26821151
5. Howell MD, Kim BE, Gao P, Grant AV, Boguniewicz M, Debenedetto A, Schneider L, Beck LA, Barnes KC, Leung DY. Cytokine modulation of atopic dermatitis filaggrin skin expression. *J Allergy Clin Immunol*. 2007 Jul;120(1):150–155. doi: 10.1016/j.jaci.2007.04.031. Epub 2007 May 23. PMID: 17512043
6. Silverberg JI. Association between adult atopic dermatitis, cardiovascular disease, and increased heart attacks in three population-based studies. *Allergy*. 2015 Oct;70(10):1300–1308. doi: 10.1111/all.12685. Epub 2015 Aug 6. PMID: 26148129
7. Kim JE, Kim HS. Microbiome of the skin and gut in atopic dermatitis (AD): Understanding the pathophysiology and finding novel management strategies. *J Clin Med*. 2019 Apr 2;8(4):444. doi: 10.3390/jcm8040444. PMID: 30987008
8. Nyangahu DD, Jaspan HB. Influence of maternal microbiota during pregnancy on infant immunity. *Clin Exp Immunol*. 2019 Oct;198(1):47–56. doi: 10.1111/cei.13331. Epub 2019 Jun 21. PMID: 31121057
9. Romano-Keeler J, Weitkamp JH. Maternal influences on fetal microbial colonization and immune development. *Pediatr Res*. 2015 Jan;77(1–2):189–195. doi: 10.1038/pr.2014.163. Epub 2014 Oct 13. PMID: 25310759

10. Amenyogbe N, Kollmann TR, Ben-Othman R Early-Life Host-Microbiome Interphase: The Key Frontier for Immune Development. *Front Pediatr.* 2017 May 24;5:111. doi: 10.3389/fped.2017.00111. eCollection 2017. PMID: 28596951

11. Vuillermin PJ, Macia L, Nanan R, Tang ML, Collier F, Brix S. The maternal microbiome during pregnancy and allergic disease in the offspring. *Semin Immunopathol.* 2017 Nov;39(6):669–675. doi: 10.1007/s00281-017-0652-y. Epub 2017 Oct 16. PMID: 29038841

12. Belkaid Y, Segre JA. Dialogue between skin microbiota and immunity. *Science.* 2014 Nov 21;346(6212):954–959. doi: 10.1126/science.1260144. PMID: 25414304

13. Francuzik W, Franke K, Schumann RR, Heine G, Worm M. Propionibacterium acnes abundance correlates inversely with Staphylococcus aureus: Data from Atopic dermatitis skin microbiome. *Acta Derm Venereol.* 2018 Apr 27;98(5):490–495. doi: 10.2340/00015555-2896. PMID: 29379979

14. Kong HH, Oh J, Deming C, Conlan S, Grice EA, Beatson MA, Nomicos E, Polley EC, Komarow HD. NISC Comparative Sequence Program, Murray PR, Turner ML, Segre JA. Temporal shifts in the skin microbiome associated with disease flares and treatment in children with atopic dermatitis. *Genome Res.* 2012 May;22(5):850–859. doi: 10.1101/gr.131029.111. Epub 2012 Feb 6. PMID: 22310478

15. Costello EK, Lauber CL, Hamady M, Fierer N, Gordon JI, Knight R. Bacterial community variation in human body habitats across space and time. *Science* 2009 Dec 18;326(5960):1694–1697. doi: 10.1126/science.1177486. Epub 2009 Nov 5. PMID: 19892944

16. Hon KL, Tsang YC, Pong NH, *et al.* Exploring Staphylococcus epidermidis in atopic eczema: friend or foe?. *Clin Exp Dermatol.* 2016 Aug;41(6):659–63. doi: 10.1111/ced.12866. PMID: 27416972

17. Paller AS, Kong HH, Seed P, Naik S, Scharschmidt TC, Gallo RL, Luger T, Irvine AD. The microbiome in patients with atopic dermatitis. *J Allergy Clin Immunol.* 2019 Jan;143(1):26–35. doi: 10.1016/j.jaci.2018.11.015. Epub 2018 Nov 23. PMID: 30476499

18. Wilson SR, Thé L, Batia LM, Beattie K, Katibah GE, McClain SP, Pellegrino M, Estandian DM, Bautista DM. The epithelial cell-derived atopic dermatitis cytokine TSLP activates neurons to induce itch. *Cell.* 2013 Oct 10;155(2):285–295. doi: 10.1016/j.cell.2013.08.057. Epub 2013 Oct 3. PMID: 24094650

19. Penders J, Thijs C, van den Brandt PA, Kummeling I, Snijders B, Stelma F, Adams H, van Ree R, Stobberingh EE. Gut microbiota composition and development of atopic manifestations in infancy: the KOALA Birth Cohort Study.

Gut. 2007 May;56(5):661–667. doi: 10.1136/gut.2006.100164. Epub 2006 Oct 17. PMID: 17047098

20. Watanabe S, Narisawa Y, Arase S, Okamatsu H, Ikenaga T, Tajiri Y, Kumemura M. Differences in fecal microflora between patients with atopic dermatitis and healthy control subjects. *J Allergy Clin Immunol.* 2003 Mar;111(3):587–591. doi: 10.1067/mai.2003.105. PMID: 12642841

21. Fujimura KE, Sitarik AR, Havstad S, Lin DL, Levan S, Fadrosh D, Panzer AR, LaMere B, Rackaityte E, Lukacs NW, Wegienka G, Boushey HA, Ownby DR, Zoratti EM, Levin AM, Johnson CC, Lynch SV. Neonatal gut microbiota associates with childhood multisensitized atopy and T cell differentiation. *Nat Med.* 2016 Oct;22(10):1187–1191. doi: 10.1038/nm.4176. Epub 2016 Sep 12. PMID: 27618652

22. Romagnani S. Regulation of the T cell response. *Clin Exp Allergy.* 2006 Nov;36(11):1357–66. doi: 10.1111/j.1365-2222.2006.02606.x. PMID: 17083345

23. Groux H, O'Garra A, Bigler M, Rouleau M, Antonenko S, de Vries JE, Roncarolo MG. A CD4+ T-cell subset inhibits antigen-specific T-cell responses and prevents colitis. *Nature* 1997 Oct 16;389(6652):737–742. doi: 10.1038/39614. PMID: 9338786

24. Makrgeorgou A, Leonardi-Bee J, Bath-Hextall FJ, Murrell DF, Tang ML, Roberts A, Boyle RJ. Probiotics for treating eczema. *Cochrane Database Syst Rev.* 2018 Nov 21;11(11):CD006135. doi: 10.1002/14651858.CD006135.pub3. PMID: 30480774

25. Reiger M, Traidl-Hoffmann C, Neumann AU. The skin microbiome as a clinical biomarker in atopic eczema: Promises, navigation, and pitfalls. *J Allergy Clin Immunol.* 2020 Jan;145(1):93–96. doi: 10.1016/j.jaci.2019.11.004. PMID: 31910987

Suggested Further Reading

Brunner PM, Leung DYM, Guttman-Yassky E. Immunologic, microbial, and epithelial interactions in atopic dermatitis. *Ann Allergy Asthma Immunol.* 2018 Jan;120(1):34–41. doi: 10.1016/j.anai.2017.09.055. Epub 2017 Nov 7. PMID: 29126710

SHI ZHEN TEA I: INSIDE LOOK AT A BOTANICAL FORMULA

Nan Yang, PhD* and Xiu-Min Li, MD, MS†

*Department of Microbiology & Immunology
†Department of Pathology, Microbiology and Immunology,
and Department of Otolaryngology
New York Medical College, Valhalla, New York 10595, USA

Abstract

Shi Zhen Tea I is a staple of Dr. Li's eczema protocol. Administered orally in capsules, it has been studied exhaustively for safety, quality, and purity and is representative of the care that the team brings to all its work.

Keywords: Botanical chemistry, product quality control, PK, and safety of TCM formulation (Shi Zhen Tea I) for eczema.

Introduction

Atopic dermatitis (AD, also known as eczema) is a chronic inflammatory skin disorder. It has a worldwide prevalence of up to 20% in children.[1] Topical corticosteroids are commonly used for AD treatment. Currently, more and more patients who have chronic atopic dermatitis choose phototherapy as an alternative to topical corticosteroids to avoid side effects of long-term topical corticosteroid use and the risk of steroid addiction.[2] A traditional Chinese medicine formula — Shi Zhen Tea I (SZT-1) — has been developed for treatment of chronic AD. In this chapter, we will discuss botanical chemistry, quality control, toxicology and clinical applications.

Botanical Chemistry

SZT-1 formula contains 9 different medicinal herbal plants, *Flos Lonicerae Japonicae* (Jin Yin Hua), *Fructurs Forsythiae Suspensae* (Lian Qiao), *Isatidis* (Qing Dai), *Radix Glycyrrhizae Uralensis* (Gan Cao), *Radix Potentillae Chinensis* (Zi Cao), *Fructus Kochia Scopariae* (Di Fu Zi), *Massa medicata* (Jian Qu, Shen Qu), *Moutan Cortex Radicis* (Dan Pi), *Poriae Cocos* (Fu Ling). The ingredients in SZT-1 formula and their biological activities are summarized below.

Chemicals for Each Herb

Flos Lonicerae Japonicae (Jin Yin Hua) has been used for several thousand years in China for its anti-bacterial,[3] anti-oxidative,[4] and anti-allergy effects.[5] More than 200 chemical constituents have been identified in *Flos Lonicerae Japonicae*, which includes iridoids loganin, ketologanin[6]; organic acids,[7] flavonoids (quercetin, rutin, uteolin), triterpenoids, and ursolic acid (limonin[8] and volatile oils[7]).

Fructus Forsythiae Suspensa (Lian Qiao) is the dried root for Forsythia suspense (Thunb.) Vahl, which was traditionally used for clearing heat and reducing swelling. It contains more than 200 compounds in which lignans are the major components. Forsythialan A and forsythialan B showed antioxidant and anti-inflammatory effects,[9] while matairesinol showed anti-allergic effects.[10] Other compounds such as flavonoids (rutin, hesperidin, hyperin, or quercetin), terpenoids, cyclohexylethanol derivatives, and alkaloids were also isolated from this plant.

Indigo naturalis (Qing Dai) was traditionally processed and obtained from *Strobilanthes cusia* or *Isatis tinctorial*. It contains indigo, indirubin, and tryptanthrin, etc., which showed anti-tumor,[11] immunodulation, and anti-inflammatory effects.[12,13]

Radix Arnebia (Zi Cao) is the dried root of Arnebia euchroma, which has been traditionally used for skin wounds[14]. Its major constituents are Shikonin,[15] alkannin,[16] and isohexenylnaphthazarin.[17]

Radix Glycyrrhizae Uralensis (Gan Cao) is one of the most commonly used herbs in traditional Chinese medicine. It contains many chemical constituents, such as treiterpene glycosides (glycyrrhizin), chalocones (isoliquiritigenin and isoliquiritin), and flavanones (liquiritigenin and liquiritin).[18]

Fructus Kochia Scopariae (Di Fu Zi) is the fruit of Kochia scoparia (L.) Schrad. It has a long usage history as a traditional Chinese medicine with more than 100 identified compounds. The main active compounds are triterpenoids (Momordin Ic, which has been shown for its anti-inflammatory effect).[19] Flavonoids (such as glucopyranose, rhamnose) are other major components. Carbohydrates, amino acids, organic acid, essential oils, and heterocyclics were also found.

Massa medicata (Jian Qu, Shen Qu) was traditionally used to strengthen the gut and spleen and improve digestion. Several galactosyl acylaglycerols and benzochroman were identified from *massa medicate fromentatata*.[20] In vitro study showed that benzochroman significantly inhibited LPS stimulated IL-6 production in bone marrow-derived dendritic cells.[20]

Moutan cortex radicis (Dan Pi) is the root bark of *Paeonia suffruticosa Andrews*. Traditionally, it was used as a treatment for promoting blood circulation and reducing excessive heat from the blood. Researchers have identified more than 100 chemical constituents in this herbal medicine. The major constituents are Monoterpene glycosides (paeoniflorin) and phenols (paeonol). It was found that paeonol has anti-inflammatory effects.[21]

Poriae cocos (Fu Ling) is a saprophytic fungus that has been used as a traditional Chinese medicine for its diuretic effect and immunity-strengthening effect. The major components in it are triterpenoids such as tumulosic acid and poricoic acid[22,23] and polysaccharides.[24,25]

Quality Control

Medicinal herbs normally contain hundreds of chemical constituents. Many of these ingredients have been shown to have different therapeutic effects. Quality control for traditional Chinese medicine is very critical. It is directly linked to efficacy and safety. Herb quality can be affected by many factors, such as the plant origin, growth method, and environmental conditions, local climate, harvest location and season, processing methods, and storage conditions. The formulation of traditional Chinese medicine is even more complicated than for individual herbs. No single active compound or several compounds can represent the overall effect of a formula. Normally, identified bioactive compounds can be selected as indicators for quality control. Standardized quality-control methods for the raw herbal materials used and the final commercial product are required to establish safety and medicinal efficacy.

SZT-1 formula was manufactured in a modern factory using classical herbology and Good Manufacturing Practices (GMP) standards. Each raw herbal medicine was first inspected and identified by botanists trained in Traditional Chinese Herbology for authentication, then its High Performance Liquid Chromatography (HPLC) fingerprint examined for chemical constituents, and finally biological activities of the herbal product were tested in vitro. In addition, the manufacturing protocol was standardized and chromatographic fingerprinting was used to monitor the processing procedures and the quality of different batch of final products.

Method

Each herb used in the preparation of the SZT-1 formula meets the standards in Pharmacopoeia of the People's Republic of China. We have also developed HPLC method to qualitatively and quantitatively evaluate the quality of SZT-1 formula in order to obtain consistent results. The HPLC fingerprint of SZT-1 is shown in Fig. 7.1. The HPLC method has high reproducibility and high accuracy. A total of 26 diagnostic peaks were observed. The individual peak was characterized by comparison of its retention time, peak intensity, and the UV spectra.

The overall evaluation of the quality of herbal medicines must include their pharmacological effects. The therapeutic effect of herbal medicine is based on the active components presented in it. Several separation and purification methods, such as liquid-liquid extraction, preparative HPLC, and thin-layer

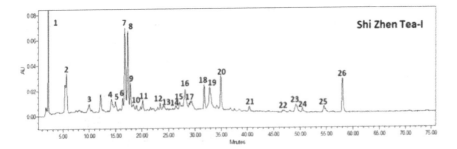

Figure 7.1.   HPLC fingerprint for Shi Zhen Tea-1

chromatography, were used to isolate individual compounds. These compounds were then characterized for chemical properties using UV (ultraviolet spectrometry), LC-MS (Mass spectrometry), and NMR (nuclear magnetic resonance spectrometry), etc. Identified chemical components will then be used as chemical markers, and quantitatively analyzed using our developed HPLC method.

Atopic dermatitis is a very complex disease. There is no in vitro model that can adequately reflect all its elements. Therefore, we have established combined in vitro experiments that include analysis of the inhibitory effect on IgE, TNF-alpha, and eotaxin on different cells lines to test bioactivity of the identified compounds, the quality of raw herbal materials, and the potency of the whole formula. The efficacy and quality of the herbal medicine were fully evaluated and ensured by comparing the bioactivities of different batches of the raw herbal materials and the SZT-1 formula.

The microbial contamination, heavy metals, and pesticide residues of each herb and the final product were analyzed on GC-MS and atomic absorption by certified third-party companies to ensure the safety of the raw herbs and to meet quality and safety standards of the FDA of the US. Only those raw materials meeting current US standards of safety for food products will be used for production.

Safety Study in Animal Models

Historical Use of Individual Herbal Components

All 9 herbal medicines used in SZT-1 formula are safe and have long usage history in China. Database searching showed no reports of toxicity directly linked to the usage of these 9 herbs at their therapeutic dosages.

In Vivo Experiment of SZT-1

To further ensure the safety of the formula, we tested the SZT-1 formula on mice following two protocols: acute safety and chronic safety assay. We monitored those mice for an additional 2 weeks. In the acute safety experiment, no animal deaths occurred after feeding 10 times normal daily dose (127 mg/day) and no abnormal behavior or diarrhea was observed in 14 days. No abnormalities of major organs were detected by histological analysis. In the chronic safety assay, mice were fed with 5 times of the normal daily dose (63.5mg/day) for 14 consecutive days. All mice appeared

Table 7.1.   Acute and chronic toxicity levels; blood counts in mouse studies.

Treatment	Dose	Time	Death (12 hrs)	Death (2 weeks)	Morbidity Percentage	Mortality Percentage
Acute toxicity Sham	10X	1 day	0/5	0/5	0	0
Shi Zhen Tea-1	10X	1 day	0/5	0/5	0	0
Sub-Chronic toxicity Sham	5X	14 days	0/5	0/5	0	0
Shi Zhen Tea -1	5X	14 days	0/5	0/5	0	0

CBC Testing

Biochemical Assays

	White Blood Cells (103/mL)	Red Blood Cells (106/mL)	Hemoglobin (g/dl)	Platelets (103/mL)	Neutrophils	Lymphocytes	Eosinophils	Basophils	BUN (mg/dL)	ALT (U/L)
Naive	7.6 ± 1.9	9.6 ± 0.8	15.3 ± 0.8	1252.8 ± 278.2	1515.6 ± 231.3	5705.6 ± 1887.0	167.2 ± 102.6	65.8 ± 38.7	21.0 ± 3.9	26.8 ± 5.3
SZT 1	5.3 ± 1.5	10.2 ± 0.6	16.3 ± 1.2	1455.6 ± 429.1	1764.2 ± 690.9	3248.6 ± 925.9	176.2 ± 114.7	50.2 ± 52.2	22.6 ± 2.6	76.8 ± 16.1
Ref	5.4~16.0	6.7~9.71	10.2~16.6	799~1300	1900~3600	8000~18000	0~500	0.0~400	9~30	16~58

healthy. Mice were sacrificed and subjected to complete blood count (CBC) and biochemical analysis of liver and kidney functions. Data showed that the white blood cell, red blood cell, hemoglobin, platelet levels, serum ALT, and BUN levels were all in the normal range as the control group (Table 7.1). All these data showed that SZT-1 formula has a large therapeutic safety profile.

References

1. Nutten S. Atopic dermatitis: global epidemiology and risk factors. *Ann Nutr Metab.* 2015;66(Suppl 1):8–16.
2. Chong M, Fonacier L. Treatment of eczema: Corticosteroids and beyond. *Clin Rev Allergy Immunol.* 2016;51:249–262.
3. Han J, *et al.* Comparison of anti-bacterial activity of three types of di-O-caffeoylquinic acids in Lonicera japonica flowers based on microcalorimetry. *Chin J Nat Med.* 2014;12:108–113.
4. Tang D, Li HJ, Chen J, Guo CW, Li P. Rapid and simple method for screening of natural antioxidants from Chinese herb Flos Lonicerae Japonicae by DPPH-HPLC-DAD-TOF/MS. *J Sep Sci.*2008;31:3519–3526.
5. Oku H, Ogawa Y, Iwaoka E, Ishiguro K. Allergy-preventive effects of chlorogenic acid and iridoid derivatives from flower buds of Lonicera japonica. *Biol Pharm Bull.* 2011;34:1330–1333.
6. Yang R, *et al.* Separation of five iridoid glycosides from *Lonicerae Japonicae* Flos Using high-speed counter-current chromatography and their anti-inflammatory and antibacterial activities. *Molecules.* 2019; 24:197.
7. Cai H, *et al.* Profiling and characterization of volatile components from non-fumigated and sulfur-fumigated Flos Lonicerae Japonicae using comprehensive two-dimensional gas chromatography time-of-flight mass spectrometry coupled with chemical group separation. *Molecules.* 2018;18:1368–1382.
8. Fang Z, Li J, Yang R, Fang L, Zhang Y. A review: The Triterpenoid saponins and biological activities of *Lonicera Linn. Molecules.* 2020;25:3773.
9. Piao XL, Jang MH, Cui J, Piao X. Lignans from the fruits of Forsythia suspensa. *Bioorg Med Chem Lett.* 2008;18:1980–1984.
10. Sung YY, Lee AY, Kim HK. Forsythia suspensa fruit extracts and the constituent matairesinol confer anti-allergic effects in an allergic dermatitis mouse model. *J Ethnopharmacol.* 2016;187:49–56.

11. Chang HN, *et al.* Indigo naturalis and its component tryptanthrin exert anti-angiogenic effect by arresting cell cycle and inhibiting Akt and FAK signaling in human vascular endothelial cells. *J Ethnopharmacol.* 2015;174:474–481.

12. Kawai S, *et al.* Indigo Naturalis ameliorates murine dextran sodium sulfate-induced colitis via aryl hydrocarbon receptor activation. *J Gastroenterol.* 2017;52:904–919.

13. Suzuki H, *et al.* Therapeutic efficacy of the Qing Dai in patients with intractable ulcerative colitis. *World J Gastroenterol.*2013;19:2718–2722.

14. Nasiri E, *et al.* The healing effect of arnebia euchroma ointment versus silver sulfadiazine on burn wounds in rat. *World J Plast Surg.* 2015;4:134–144.

15. Liu T, *et al.* Optimization of shikonin homogenate extraction from Arnebia euchroma using response surface methodology. *Molecules.* 2013;18:466–481.

16. Yoshihisa Y, *et al.* Alkannin, HSP70 inducer, protects against UVB-induced apoptosis in human keratinocytes. *PLoS One.* 2012;7:e47903.

17. Damianakos H, *et al.* Antimicrobial and cytotoxic isohexenylnaphthazarins from Arnebia euchroma (Royle) Jonst. (Boraginaceae) callus and cell suspension culture. *Molecules.* 2012;17:14310–14322.

18. Li F, *et al.* Review of constituents and biological activities of triterpene saponins from Glycyrrhizae Radix et Rhizoma and its solubilization characteristics. *Molecules.* 2020;25:3904.

19. Yoo SR, *et al.* Quantification analysis and in vitro anti-inflammatory effects of 20-hydroxyecdysone, momordin Ic, and oleanolic acid from the fructus of Kochia scoparia. *Pharmacogn Mag.* 2017;13:339–344.

20. Sun YN, *et al.* Isolation and identification of benzochroman and acylglycerols from Massa Medicata Fermentata and their inhibitory effects on LPS-stimulated cytokine production in bone marrow-derived dendritic cells. *Molecules.* 2018;23:2400.

21. Fu PK, *et al.* Anti-inflammatory and anticoagulative effects of paeonol on LPS-induced acute lung injury in rats. *Evid Based Complement Alternat Med.* 2012:837513.

22. Chao CL, *et al.* The lanostane triterpenoids in *Poria cocos* play beneficial roles in immunoregulatory activity. *Life (Basel).* 2021;11:111.

23. Ukiya M, *et al.* Inhibition of tumor-promoting effects by poricoic acids G and H and other lanostane-type triterpenes and cytotoxic activity of poricoic acids A and G from Poria cocos. *J Nat Prod.* 2002;65:462–465.

24. Li CY, *et al.* Inhibition of calcium oxalate formation and antioxidant activity of carboxymethylated *Poria cocos* polysaccharides. *Oxid Med Cell Longev.* 2021:6653593.

25. Wang D, *et al.* comparative studies on polysaccharides, triterpenoids, and essential oil from fermented mycelia and cultivated sclerotium of a medicinal and edible mushroom, Poria cocos. *Molecules.* 2000;25:1269.

COMPUTATIONAL APPROACHES TO REVEAL THE ACTIVE COMPOUNDS AND MOLECULAR TARGETS FROM TCM FORMULAS FOR ECZEMA

Zhen-Zhen Wang, PhD

Academy of Chinese Medical Science, Henan University of Chinese Medicine, Zhengzhou 450046, China
Department of Microbiology and Immunology, New York Medical College, New York 10595, USA

Abstract

Traditional Chinese Medicine (TCM) has shown significant success in treating eczema by improving skin lesions, itching, sleeping loss, and facilitating reduction of topical steroids and antihistamines used in pediatric and adult patients with severe eczema. However, the biological mechanisms of TCM are extremely elusive due to the presence of multiple active compounds in herbs and their unknown metabolites. The recent development of cheminformatics and bioinformatics provides powerful tools to investigate the multi-components-multi-targets system in TCM. By predicting and enriching new actionable targets for numerous compounds, computational approaches including but not limited to systems pharmacology, in silico molecular docking, and molecular dynamics simulation give insight into the active compounds, molecular targets, and biological function of TCM for the treatment of eczema.

Keywords: Cheminformatics, bioinformatics, systems pharmacology, in silico molecular docking, molecular dynamics simulation

Introduction

TCM has a history of thousands of years of use in Asia.[1] In recent years, many compounds have been separated from the herbs and formulas that comprise the TCM formulary and their structure and pharmacological activities have been identified. Numerous drugs for diverse diseases on the market have been discovered based on original structure or derivatives of active compounds from TCM, such as artemisinin[2] and salicylic acid.[3] We have learned that apart from the active compounds, most molecules separated from herbs are ineffective with poor pharmacological action. Researchers have wasted copious resources investigating these molecules by trial and error, and the progress of drug discovery has been slowed. Direct discovery of new drugs is complicated by the fact that TCM is viewed as system medicine, and the efficacy of TCM derives from synergistic effects of multiple active compounds from different herbs. It is a major challenge to distinguish the molecular and biological mechanisms that play crucial roles in efficacy from those that play supporting roles, and those that do nothing. However, with the development of bioinformatics and cheminformatics,[4,5] new technology including high-throughput genomic sequencing, proteomics, machine learning, and computational simulation make it possible to collect and predict the potential targets of numerous compounds in TCM for the treatment of diseases. The system network is a powerful tool to select the highly connected components as hubs, which help to uncover the active compounds, biological targets, and molecular mechanisms of TCM formulas for the treatment of eczema. Instead of random testing, computational approaches not only provide a solution to solve multi-components and multi-targets problems in TCM but might also significantly reduce the time and cost in drug discovery.

General Procedures

The general workflow of computational strategies is shown in Fig. 8.1. The representative online databases are listed in Table 8.1. The active compounds are usually selected based on specific criteria from TCM compound databases such as TCM Systems Pharmacology (TCMSP),[6] TCM@Taiwan,[7] and Batman-TCM[8] (Table 8.1). The selection criteria depend on vital properties of compounds as available drugs such as oral bioavailability (OB) and drug-likeness (DL). OB represents the percentage that is absorbed into the system from an orally administered dose of drugs. DL stands for the similarity of given compound with the physiochemical or/and structural properties of existing drugs, which have been used to evaluate a drug's potential. In addition, some compounds in herbs published with poor physicochemical properties but excellent pharmacological activities also need to be taken into consideration.

Compounds with diverse structures have been investigated for multiple targets using high-throughput technologies in the progress of drug-discovery, which provide the opportunity to predict the cheminformatic target of the unknown compounds based on the structures.[9] Thus, the targets of active compounds are collected based on predicted algorithms or experimental validation from self-established models or online databases such as HitPick,[10] Swiss Target Prediction,[11] Similarity Ensemble Approach (SEA),[12] PubChem,[13] and DrugBank[14] (Table 8.1). Moreover, the genes or proteins related to the pathological process of eczema are obtained from integrated databases such as Therapeutic Target Database (TTD),[15] Genetic Association Database,[16] GeneCards,[17] and Open Targets Platform[18] (Table 8.1). The shared genes or proteins between active compounds and eczema are considered as biological targets of TCM for the regulation and treatment of eczema. Then, with the identification of these targets, analysis in different levels can be conducted to reveal the pharmacological mechanism of action for TCM. By target enrichment, the significant Gene Ontology (GO) terms and KEGG pathways can be acquired through online databases such as DAVID[19] or KOBAS[20] to help elucidate the biologically comprehensive regulation of TCM at the cellular, tissue, and organ levels. In addition, protein-protein interaction datasets have been investigated by a large number of

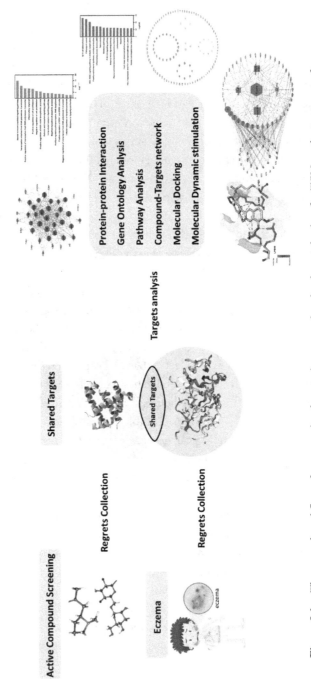
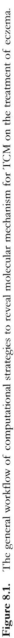

Figure 8.1.   The general workflow of computational strategies to reveal molecular mechanism for TCM on the treatment of eczema.

Table 8.1. Representative list of online databases used in computational strategies.

Functions	Database Name	Website
Active Compounds Screening from TCM	TCMSP[1]	lsp.nwu.edu.cn/tcmsp.php
	TCM@Taiwan[2]	tcm.cmu.edu.tw/index.php
	BATMAN-TCM[3]	bionet.ncpsb.org/batman-tcm/
	TCM-MESH[4]	mesh.tcm.microbioinformatics.org/
	TCMID[5]	megabionet.org/tcmid/
Targets Collection for Active Compounds	Drugbank[6]	drugbank.ca/
	SEA[7]	sea.bkslab.org/
	SwissTarget Prediction[8]	swisstargetprediction.ch/
	PubChem[9]	pubchem.ncbi.nlm.nih.gov
	HitPick[10]	mips.helmholtz-muenchen.de/hitpick/cgi-bin/index.cgi?content=targetPrediction.html
	SuperPred[11]	prediction.charite.de/
	ChemMapper[12]	lilab-ecust.cn/chemmapper/index.html
	PharmMapper[13]	lilab-ecust.cn/pharmmapper/
Targets Collection for Eczema	TTD[14]	db.idrblab.org/ttd/
	Genetic Association Database[15]	geneticassociationdb.nih.gov
	GeneCards[16]	genecards.org
	Open Targets Platform[17]	platform.opentargets.org/
	DisGeNET[18]	disgenet.org/web/DisGeNET/menu/home
	GEO[19]	ncbi.nlm.nih.gov/geo/
Targets Enrichment	DAVID[20]	david.ncifcrf.gov/
	KOBAS[21]	kobas.cbi.pku.edu.cn
	NetworkAnalyst[22]	networkanalyst.ca
Protein-Protein Interaction	String[22]	https://www.string-db.org/

experimental and computational methods, which has become a key method to predict gene function, and discover disease genes.[21] With shared targets, protein-protein interaction networks can be easily established using online databases such as String,[22] providing insight into the targets functions and correlations. The different types of networks containing but not limited to

TCM formula, herbs, compounds, targets, GO terms, and pathways can be built to understand both direct and indirect interactions between components in networks. The sensitivity of network topology can be evaluated based on graph theory and statistical analysis to select highly connected components as hubs from networks.

To further evaluate the binding affinity and possibility between active compounds and targets in three-dimensional models, molecular docking and molecular dynamic stimulation can be used while accounting for both compounds and protein structures.

Recently, the mechanisms and functions of numerous TCM formulas for various diseases have been investigated using computational strategies such as Run Zao Zhi Yang capsules (RZZYC),[23] Xiao Feng San (XFS),[24] and anti-asthma herbal medicine intervention (ASHMI)[25]. In addition, we performed computational analysis on Shi Zhen Tea I (SZT) using computational approaches, including ADME evaluation, herb feature mapping, drug target mining, network and pathway analyses, and molecular docking. SZT is a derivative of XFS that has been developed by our group and successfully used in the US as integrative eczema therapy.[26] Fifty-one compounds including flavonoid, alkaloid, phenylpropanoid, terpene, and steroid have been identified sharing 81 potential biological targets for the treatment of eczema. The efficacy of SZT in eczema may be attributed to immune and metabolic functions via regulation of multiple pathways and networks such as Th17 cell differentiation, pathways in cancer, metabolic pathways, and PI3K-Akt signaling pathway.[27]

Conclusion and Future Perspective

Eczema is a chronic inflammatory skin disease impacted by environmental factors, infections, immune disorders, and deficiencies in skin barrier function. TCM has demonstrated excellent efficacy in treating eczema without serious adverse effects by regulating the immune system and rebuilding the skin barrier. The computational strategies describing the multi-compounds-multi-targets synergy of TCM on eczema give direct insight into potential mechanisms of TCM in molecular levels.

Network pharmacology was initially put forward to investigate polypharmacological activities of drugs and reveal the synergism law of multi-component drugs.[28] The development of high-throughput technologies and computational modeling further increase the reliability of network pharmacology analysis. With the development of genomic or proteomics technology, genetic characteristics of individual patient can be detected, which might give the opportunity to achieve personalized and precision TCM treatment. However, the compounds in herbs and their effective concentration are not in consideration. The lack of quantitative and dynamic relationships between network nodes is the major limitation of computational approaches. Quantitative systems pharmacology might increase the precision and guide the analysis of TCM components in the future. Ultimately, the predicted active compounds, targets, and mechanisms of TCM still need to be validated through in vivo and in vitro study.

References

1. Wang Z, Wang ZZ, Geliebter J, Tiwari R, Li XM. Traditional Chinese medicine for food allergy and eczema *Ann Allergy Asthma Immunol.* 2021;126(6): 639–654.
2. Tu Y. The discovery of artemisinin (qinghaosu) and gifts from Chinese medicine. *Nat Med.* 2011;17(10):1217–1220.
3. Rivas-San Vicente M, Plasencia J. Salicylic acid beyond defence: Its role in plant growth and development. *J Exp Bot.* 2011;62(10):3321–3338.
4. Guha R, Bender A. *Computational Approaches in Cheminformatics and Bioinformatics.* John Wiley & Sons, Inc., 2012.
5. Birtwistle MR, Hansen J, Gallo JM, Muppirisetty S, Schlessinger A. Systems pharmacology: An overview. In *Systems Pharmacology and Pharmacodynamics.* Springer International Publishing, 2016, pp 53–80.
6. Ru J, Li P, Wang J, Zhou W, Li B, Huang C, Guo Z, Tao W, Yang Y, Xu X, Li Y, Wang Y, Yang L. TCMSP: A database of systems pharmacology for drug discovery from herbal medicines. *J Cheminform.* 2014;6:13.
7. Chen CY. TCM Database@Taiwan: The world's largest traditional Chinese medicine database for drug screening in silico. *PLoS One.* 2011;6(1):e15939.
8. Liu Z, Guo F, Wang Y, Li C, Zhang X, Li H, Diao L, Gu J, Wang W, Li D, He F. BATMAN-TCM: A bioinformatics analysis tool for molecular mechanism of traditional Chinese medicine. *Sci Rep.* 2016;6:21146.
9. Nikolic K, Mavridis L, Bautista-Aguilera OM, Marco-Contelles J, Stark H, do Carmo Carreiras M, Rossi I, Massarelli P, Agbaba D, Ramsay RR, Mitchell JB.

Predicting targets of compounds against neurological diseases using cheminformatic methodology. *J Comput Aided Mol Des.* 2015;29(2):183–198.

10. Liu X, Vogt I, Haque T, Campillos M. HitPick: A web server for hit identification and target prediction of chemical screenings. *Bioinformatics.* 2013;29(15):1910–1912.

11. Daina A, Michielin O, Zoete V. SwissTargetPrediction: Updated data and new features for efficient prediction of protein targets of small molecules. *Nucleic Acids Res.* 2019, *47* (W1), W357–W364.

12. Keiser MJ, *et al.* Relating protein pharmacology by ligand chemistry. *Nat Biotechnol.* 2007;25(2):197–206.

13. Kim S, Chen J, Cheng T, Gindulyte A, He J, He S, Li Q, Shoemaker BA, Thiessen PA, Yu B, Zaslavsky L, Zhang J, Bolton EE. PubChem 2019 update: improved access to chemical data. *Ncleic Acids Res.* 2019;47(D1): D1102–D1109.

14. Wishart DS, Knox C, Guo AC, Cheng D, Shrivastava S, Tzur D, Gautam B, Hassanali M. DrugBank: A knowledgebase for drugs, drug actions and drug targets. *Nucleic Acids Res.* 2008;36:D901–D906.

15. Wang Y, Zhang S, Li F, Zhou Y, Zhang Y, Wang Z, Zhang R, Zhu J, Ren Y, Tan Y, Qin C, Li Y, Li X, Chen Y, Zhu F. Therapeutic target database 2020: Enriched resource for facilitating research and early development of targeted therapeutics. *Nucleic Acids Res.* 2020;48(D1):D1031–D1041.

16. Becker KG, Barnes KC, Bright TJ, Wang SA. The genetic association database. *Nat Genet.* 2004;36:431–432.

17. Safran M, Solomon I, Shmueli O, Lapidot M, Shen-Orr S, Adato A, Ben-Dor U, Esterman N, Rosen N, Peter I, Olender T, Chalifa-Caspi V, Lancet D. GeneCards 2002: Towards a complete, object-oriented, human gene compendium. *Bioinformatics.* 2002;18(11):1542–1543.

18. Carvalho-Silva D, Pierleoni A, Pignatelli M, Ong C, Fumis L, Karamanis N, Carmona M, Faulconbridge A, Hercules A, McAuley E, Miranda A, Peat G, Spitzer M, Barrett J, Hulcoop DG, Papa E, Koscielny G, Dunham I. Open Targets Platform: New developments and updates two years on. *Nucleic Acids Res.* 2019;47(D1):D1056–D1065.

19. Huang DW, *et al.* Systematic and integrative analysis of large gene lists using DAVID bioinformatics resources. *Nat Protoc.* 2009;4(1):44–57.

20. Xie C, *et al.* KOBAS 2.0: A web server for annotation and identification of enriched pathways and diseases. *Nucleic Acids Res.* 2011;39(Web Server issue): W316–3122.

21. Kotlyar M, Pastrello C, Rossos A, Jurisica I. *Protein–Protein Interaction Databases.* Reference Module in Materials Science and Materials Engineering: 2018.

22. Szklarczyk D, Gable AL, Lyon D, Junge A, Wyder S, Huerta-Cepas J, Simonovic M, Doncheva NT, Morris JH, Bork P, Jensen LJ, Mering CV. STRING v11: Protein-protein association networks with increased coverage, supporting functional discovery in genome-wide experimental datasets. *Nucleic Acids Res.* 2019;47(D1):D607–D613.

23. Huang D, Chen K, Zhang FR, Yang S, Guo Q, Xu JH, Li H, Tan GZ, Yang BQ, Lu QJ, Zheng J, Li LF, Gu H. Efficacy and safety of Run Zao Zhi Yang capsule on chronic eczema: a multiple-center, randomized, double-blind, placebo-controlled clinical study. *J Dermatolog Treat.* 2019;30(7):677–684.

24. Lin YH, Chen YC, Hu S, Chen HY, Chen JL, Yang SH. Identifying core herbal treatments for urticaria using Taiwan's nationwide prescription database. *J Ethnopharmacol.* 2013;148(2):556–562.

25. Zhou W, Chen Z, Li W, Wang Y, Li X, Yu H, Ran P, Liu Z. Systems pharmacology uncovers the mechanisms of anti-asthma herbal medicine intervention (ASHMI) for the prevention of asthma. *Journal of Functional Foods.* 2019;52:611–619.

26. Thanik E, Wisniewski JA, Nowak-Wegrzyn A, Sampson H, Li XM. Effect of traditional Chinese medicine on skin lesions and quality of life in patients with moderate to severe eczema. *Ann Allergy Asthma Immunol.* 2018;121(1):135–136.

27. Wang ZZ, Jia Y, Srivastava KD, Huang W, Tiwari R, Nowak-Wegrzyn A, Geliebter J, Miao M, Li XM. Systems pharmacology and in silico docking analysis uncover association of CA2, PPARG, RXRA, and VDR with the mechanisms underlying the Shi Zhen Tea formula effect on eczema. *Evid Based Complement Alternat Med.* 2021;2021:8406127. DOI: 10.1155/2021/8406127 From NLM.

28. Hopkins AL. Network pharmacology. *Nat Biotechnol.* 2007;25(10):1110–1111.

Chapter

9

TOPICAL STEROID WITHDRAWAL

Belinda Sheary, MD*

Topical Steroid Withdrawal in 2021: Where Are We?

Topical steroid withdrawal (TSW) is a potential adverse effect of increasing amounts and/or potencies of topical steroids,[1] typically by patients being treated for atopic dermatitis (eczema).[2–5] After stopping use of topical steroids, affected patients develop new features that are not associated with their original skin condition.[1–5] Symptoms include widespread red skin, burning pain, excessive skin exfoliation, oozing skin, increased skin sensitivity, and swelling (often around their eyes or ankles).[1–6] Clinical signs include the headlight sign[2–4] (clear nose on red face), red sleeve[4,5] (redness to either the arms or legs ending abruptly at the wrist or side of foot), and/or elephant wrinkles[4] (thickened skin with reduced elasticity, commonly seen to the extensor elbow and front of knees).

TSW has been referred to by different names over time and around the world. Cases of topical steroid overuse leading to "addiction" were identified in the 1970s,[7–9] while the condition was first called "red skin syndrome"[2] and "red burning skin syndrome"[3] in the 2000s. The term "topical steroid

---

*Dr. Belinda Sheary is a general practitioner in Sydney, Australia. She completed her medical degree at the University of Newcastle and obtained her Fellowship of the Royal Australian College of General Practitioners in 2007. Dr. Sheary has a special interest in topical steroid withdrawal, and she has published a number of research papers on this topic since 2016.

withdrawal"[1] has been favored more recently over the more emotive "topical steroid addiction,"[5] while Indian dermatologists prefer "topical steroid damaged/dependent face".[10]

Risk factors for TSW include being atopic,[1-6] a history of applying potent topical steroids to the face,[1,4,6] and use of oral steroids for skin symptoms.[4,6] Females appear to be overrepresented in settings where topical steroids are misused for cosmetic purposes (for example skin lightening in Africa and Asia).[10-15] However, where TSW is associated with overuse of prescribed topical steroids, males and females are affected more equally.[4] TSW has been reported more often in adults than in children.[1,4]

The underlying mechanisms for the symptoms and signs seen in TSW are unclear, though theories have been proposed. Rapaport and Rapaport have examined the role of nitric oxide causing excessive dilatation of blood vessels giving rise to red skin,[2] while Fukaya's research focused on possible cortisol deficiency in the epidermis.[16] Cortisol is the body's own cortisone and reduces inflammation.

TSW is considered controversial and patients wanting to stop using topical steroids can struggle to find support.[17] Many doctors who acknowledge TSW maintain it is rare[18] and dismiss it as a possibility in their patients.[17] Instead, they will commonly diagnose someone with a typical history and clinical examination as having severe, untreated eczema or as having "steroid phobia".[17]

Managing TSW can be very difficult, and often patients will need to take significant time off work or study.[17] Some become unwell enough to require hospitalization.[17] Treatment is focused on symptom management.[1-3] The effectiveness of commonly used medications such as antihistamines, simple analgesia, and sleeping aids can be disappointing.[17] Options that may be more effective, such as cyclosporine,[2,3] are not readily embraced by many patients due to concerns about side effects.[17] Access to phototherapy, in addition to potential newer (and more expensive) options such as the monoclonal antibody dupilumab,[19] can be difficult.

Coping mentally with TSW is extremely challenging. Not only can symptoms last a long time (months to years) but they can also recur after being absent for significant periods of time.[6] People often find it difficult to explain to others what they are going through and can feel isolated.[17]

Depression, anxiety, and suicidal ideation have been reported.[17] Psychological support is often needed, and antidepressants are indicated in some patients.[2,3] In my research, people affected by TSW reported trying to self-manage their mental health with a variety of strategies[17] including exercising (walking, running, going to the gym, doing yoga), meditation, practicing mindfulness, doing relaxation exercises, listening to music, writing therapy, talking to a friend, praying, creating art, making jewelry, and reading self-help books.

Many people who learn about TSW online and go on to stop using their topical steroids are unprepared for the severity of subsequent symptoms and the consequent impact they have on all aspects of their life.[17] It is not surprising then, that around 30% of these people will choose to resume using topical steroids.[4,6] Some will stop using them a second time.[4,6] Less frequently acknowledged, due to difficulties with long-term follow-up, is the late resumption of topical steroid use (after 2 or more years). This is where patients, having eschewed topical steroids despite severe TSW symptoms initially, later resume their use, either briefly or regularly. This reflects the challenge these patients face in managing a chronic skin condition with few effective treatment options.

Future Directions
The Case for A Name Change

In my opinion, it is time to reconsider the terminology we use for this condition. TSW is a misnomer as use of the word "withdrawal" is inappropriate: symptoms can continue for months to years post cessation of topical steroids, and occasionally they recur after apparent "healing". While patients with worsening rashes despite escalating steroid use may resonate with the term "steroid addiction", it is not widely accepted in the medical community, and this seems unlikely to change. The "red" in "red skin syndrome" (and "red sleeve") does not reflect the experience of patients with brown and black skin who may find their affected skin is more a tan/brown/black/purple/grey color. "Topical steroid dependent face" excludes patients whose symptoms are not limited to their face in addition to those who did not apply topical steroids there.

One suggestion for a new and more appropriate name, suitable for all cases of what we now refer to as TSW, is "post steroidal syndrome".[20] Another possibility is "steroid escalating use syndrome".

Helping Existing Patients

Greater recognition of TSW in the medical community is needed so that cases of TSW can be identified readily. Accepted diagnostic criteria are essential for patients, doctors, and those researching TSW. (I proposed diagnostic criteria[4] which were published in 2018, see Appendix). Guidelines for managing TSW would assist doctors looking after these patients. Safe and effective treatments are needed to help patients with moderate to severe TSW symptoms. More research is needed to determine whether dupilumab is fit for this purpose.[19]

Prevention of Topical Steroid Withdrawal

To prevent TSW, we need to avoid topical steroid "overuse". Widespread acknowledgement of TSW may make practitioners more circumspect when prescribing them. More detailed patient education and better monitoring of patients using topical steroids have been recommended.[21] In countries such as India where topical steroids are misused for skin lightening or acne, advertising topical steroids to the general population needs to stop, as does over-the-counter access to potent and super-potent topical steroids.[14] An effective option to replace topical steroids as first-line management for eczema would be very helpful — it was hoped calcineurin inhibitors would fulfill this role, but this did not transpire.[31]

Optimizing Recommendations for Lifestyle Management of Atopic Dermatitis

To reduce the need for topical steroids, we need to ensure lifestyle recommendations for eczema management are evidence based, and any updated advice is disseminated to patients, caregivers, and relevant healthcare providers in both a clear and timely fashion. Questions we need to answer include: Which type of moisturizer is best for patients with eczema?[22] Should products with certain ingredients be avoided?[23,24] Which clothing fabrics are best?[25,26] What should we be advising about supplementation with vitamin D[27] and exposure to sunlight?[28] Can food trigger eczema flares in some patients?[29] What about other environmental factors?[30]

Reducing the Incidence of Atopic Dermatitis

If we could determine why atopic dermatitis has become more common over time and around the world,[32] we might be able to reduce the incidence of atopic dermatitis (and therefore both topical steroid use and TSW).

We need more research into preventing atopic dermatitis in at-risk infants. Unfortunately, moisturizing has been found to be ineffective for this purpose[33] and while it is thought probiotics may be useful, specific advice is currently lacking.[34] Certain early-life gut microbiomes are associated with an increased risk of developing eczema in childhood,[35] but can we prevent or modify this? If maternal stress increases the incidence of eczema in early childhood,[36,37] can we improve services to benefit the mental health of affected women, and therefore the future health of their children?

Conclusion

TSW is an adverse effect of topical steroid use which was first recognized over 40 years ago. It remains controversial and poorly acknowledged. Where topical steroids have been prescribed, it is most often seen in patients with atopic dermatitis. In Asia and Africa, TSW is more commonly seen in people who have misused topical steroids for skin lightening. As TSW is a misnomer, consideration should be given to renaming this condition. We need to do more to help patients affected by TSW and prevent new cases.

Appendix[a]

Suggested Diagnostic Criteria for TSW: A Starting Point for Discussion and Future Research

Consider TSW when the following essential criteria are fulfilled; the diagnosis becomes more likely when more of the key diagnostic criteria are also present.

---

[a] Published as part of Sheary B. Steroid withdrawal effects following long-term topical corticosteroid use. *Dermatitis.* 2018;29(4):213–218 and reprinted with permission.

Essential criteria:

1. History of long-term regular topical corticosteroids (TCS) use (months to years) where TCSs were initially effective, but over time, either increased amounts or potencies (or both) were required to reduce severity of skin symptoms
2. Itch
3. Erythema

Key diagnostic criteria:

1. History of atopy, especially atopic dermatitis
2. History of TCS use on the face, especially potent TCSs
3. History of oral prednisone use for skin symptoms
4. Burning pain on the skin
5. Skin sensitivity to previously tolerated skin products
6. Excessive skin exfoliation ("shedding")
7. Oozing skin
8. Edema, especially of the eyelids or ankles
9. "Elephant wrinkles" of the extensor elbows and anterior knees[b]
10. "Red sleeve" sign[c]

Additional supporting features that may be present:

1. Sleep disturbance
2. Mood disturbance
3. Skin pain, other than burning pain
4. Papules and pustules
5. Headlight sign

---

[b] "Elephant wrinkles": a descriptive term for apparent thickened skin with a reduction in skin elasticity, demonstrated, for example, on the anterior knees and/or extensor elbows, although not limited to these areas.

[c] "Red sleeve" sign: a descriptive term for a rebound eruption to either the upper or lower limb ending abruptly at the margin of the dorsal and palmar (or solar) border.

References

1. Hajar T, Leshem YA, Hanifin JM, *et al.* A systematic review of topical corticosteroid withdrawal ("steroid addiction") in patients with atopic dermatitis and other dermatoses. *JAAD.* 2015;72:541–549.
2. Rapaport M, Rapaport V. The red skin syndromes: corticosteroid addiction and withdrawal. *Expert Rev Dermatol.* 2006;1:547–561.
3. Rapaport MJ, Lebwohl M. Corticosteroid addiction and withdrawal in the atopic: the red burning skin syndrome. *Clin Dermatol.* 2003 May 1;21(3):201–214.
4. Sheary B. Steroid withdrawal effects following long-term topical corticosteroid use. *Dermatitis* 2018;29:213–218 doi:10.1097/DER.0000000000000387.
5. Fukaya M, Sato K, Sato M, *et al.* Topical steroid addiction in atopic dermatitis. *Drug, Healthcare and Patient Safety.* 2014;6:131–138.
6. Sheary B, Harris MF. Cessation of long-term topical steroids in adult atopic dermatitis: A prospective cohort study. *Dermatitis Contact Atopic Occup Drug.* 2020;31(5):316–320 doi: 10.1097/DER. 0000000000000602.
7. Burry JN. Topical drug addiction: Adverse effects of fluorinated corticosteroid creams and ointments. *Med J Aust.* 1973;1(8):393–396.
8. Kligman AM. Topical steroid addicts. *JAMA.* 1976 Apr 12;235(15):1550.
9. Kligman AM, Frosch PJ. Steroid addiction. *Int J Dermatol.* 1979;18:23–31.
10. Lahiri K, Coondoo A. Topical steroid damaged/dependent face (TSDF): An entity of cutaneous pharmacodependence. *Indian J Dermatol.* 2016 May;61(3):265.
11. Doss N. Topical corticosteroid abuse: Africa perspective. In: Lahiri K (eds), *A Treatise on Topical Corticosteroids in Dermatology.* Springer, Singapore, 2018. https://doi.org/10.1007/978-981-10-4609-4_23
12. Kabir Chowdhury MU. Topical corticosteroid abuse: Bangladesh perspective. In: Lahiri K (eds), *A Treatise on Topical Corticosteroids in Dermatology.* Springer, Singapore, 2018. https://doi.org/10.1007/978-981-10-4609-4_19
13. Handog EB, Enriquez-Macarayo MJ. Topical corticosteroid abuse: Southeast Asia perspective. In: Lahiri K (eds), *A Treatise on Topical Corticosteroids in Dermatology.* Springer, Singapore, 2018. https://doi.org/10.1007/978-981-10-4609-4_21
14. Jain S, Mohapatra L, Mohanty P, Jena S, Behera B. Study of clinical profile of patients presenting with topical steroid-induced facial dermatosis to a tertiary care hospital. *Indian Dermatol Online J.* 2020 Mar;11(2):208.
15. Rathi SK, D'Souza P. Abuse of topical corticosteroid as cosmetic cream: A social background of steroid dermatitis. In: Lahiri K (eds), *A Treatise on Topical*

Corticosteroids in Dermatology. Springer, Singapore, 2018 https://doi.org/10.1007/978-981-10-4609-4_12

16. Fukaya M. Histological and immunohistological findings using anti-cortisol antibody in atopic dermatitis with topical steroid addiction. *Dermatol Ther.* 2016 Mar 1;6(1):39–46.

17. Sheary B, Tyson C, Harris MF. A qualitative study exploring the views and experiences of adults who decided to cease long-term topical steroid use. *Dermatitis.* March 2, 2021;volume publish ahead of print issue. doi: 10.1097/DER.0000000000000720

18. Topical corticosteroid withdrawal. https://dermnetnz.org/topics/topical-corticosteroid-withdrawal/. Accessed 18 December, 2020.

19. Arnold KA, Treister AD, Lio PA. Dupilumab in the management of topical corticosteroid withdrawal in atopic dermatitis: A retrospective case series. *JAAD Case Reports.* 2018 Oct 1;4(9):860–862.

20. Johnson L, Tarbox M. Dr. Peter Lio discusses topical steroid addiction. *Dermatosphere.* February 22, 2021. https://podcasts.apple.com/au/podcast/dermasphere-the-dermatology-podcast/id1469274680. Accessed 24 February, 2021.

21. Hwang J, Lio PA. Topical corticosteroid withdrawal ("steroid addiction"): An update of a systematic review. *J Dermatol Treat.* 2021 Jan;27:1–24.

22. Simpson E, *et al.* Improvement of skin barrier function in atopic dermatitis patients with a new moisturizer containing a ceramide precursor. *J Dermatol Treat.* 2013 Apr 1;24(2):122–125.

23. Karagounis TK, Gittler JK, Rotemberg V, Morel KD. Use of "natural" oils for moisturization: Review of olive, coconut, and sunflower seed oil. *Pediatr Dermatol.* 2019 Jan;36(1):9–15.

24. Danby SG, Al-Enezi T, Sultan A, Chittock J, Kennedy K, Cork MJ. The effect of aqueous cream BP on the skin barrier in volunteers with a previous history of atopic dermatitis. *Br J Dermatol.* 2011 Aug;165(2):329–334.

25. Fowler Jr JF, Fowler LM, Lorenz D. Effects of merino wool on atopic dermatitis using clinical, quality of life, and physiological outcome measures. *Dermatitis.* 2019 May;30(3):198.

26. Jaros J, Wilson C, Shi VY. Fabric selection in atopic dermatitis: An evidence-based review. *Am J Clin Dermatol.* 2020 Aug;21:467–482.

27. Huang CM, Lara-Corrales I, Pope E. Effects of vitamin D levels and supplementation on atopic dermatitis: a systematic review. *Pediatr Dermatol.* 2018 Nov;35(6):754–760.

28. Byremo G, Rød G, Carlsen KH. Effect of climatic change in children with atopic eczema. *Allergy*. 2006 Dec;61(12):1403–1410.

29. Akinwande I, Salako K. Food allergies and atopic dermatitis. *InnovAiT*. 2020 Nov;13(11):655–659.

30. Kantor R, Silverberg JI. Environmental risk factors and their role in the management of atopic dermatitis. *Expert Rev Clin Immunol*. 2017 Jan 2;13(1):15–26.

31. Alomar A, Berth-Jones J, Bos JD, Giannetti A, Reitamo S, Ruzicka T, Stalder JF, Thestrup-Pedersen K, (European Working Group on Atopic Dermatitis). The role of topical calcineurin inhibitors in atopic dermatitis. *Br J Dermatol*. 2004 Dec;151:3–27.

32. Bylund S, von Kobyletzki LB, Svalstedt M, Svensson Å. Prevalence and Incidence of atopic dermatitis: A systematic review. *Acta Dermato-Venereol*. 2020 Jun 3;100.

33. Skjerven HO, Rehbinder EM, Vettukattil R, LeBlanc M, Granum B, Haugen G, Hedlin G, Landrø L, Marsland BJ, Rudi K, Sjøborg KD. Skin emollient and early complementary feeding to prevent infant atopic dermatitis (PreventADALL): A factorial, multicentre, cluster-randomised trial. *Lancet*. 2020 Mar 21;395(10228):951–961.

34. Rusu E, Enache G, Cursaru R, Alexescu A, Radu R, Onila O, Cavallioti T, Rusu F, Posea M, Jinga M, Radulian G. Prebiotics and probiotics in atopic dermatitis. *Exp Ther Med*. 2019 Aug 1;18(2):926–931.

35. Chan CW, Leung TF, Choi KC, Tsui SK, Wong CL, Chow KM, Chan JY. Association of early-life gut microbiome and lifestyle factors in the development of eczema in Hong Kong infants. *Exp Dermatol*. 2021 Jun;30(6):859–864.

36. El-Heis S, Crozier SR, Healy E, Robinson SM, Harvey NC, Cooper C, Inskip HM, Baird J, Southampton Women's Survey Study Group, Godfrey KM. Maternal stress and psychological distress preconception: association with offspring atopic eczema at age 12 months. *Clin Exp Allergy*. 2017 Jun;47(6):760–769.

37. Chan CW, Law BM, Liu YH, Ambrocio AR, Au N, Jiang M, Chow KM. The association between maternal stress and childhood eczema: a systematic review. *Int J Env Res Public Health*. 2018 Mar;15(3):395.

SUCCESSFUL MANAGEMENT OF SEVERE ECZEMA CHARACTERIZED BY CORTICOSTEROID ADDICTION AND WITHDRAWAL USING TRADITIONAL CHINESE MEDICINE

Tory McKnight, Medical Student, Clinical Researcher
and Xiu-Min Li, MD, MS

New York Medical College School of Medicine
Valhalla, New York 10595, USA

Introduction

Eczema is not exclusively an allergic condition, but rather a description of a group of conditions that cause irritation and inflammation. The most common of these in pediatric populations is the IgE antibody-mediated, allergic subtype. Allergic eczema affects 10–15% of children under the age of 5, approximately 8% of children between 6 and 7 years of age, and 7% of adolescents worldwide.[1,2] Treatment options for a person with atopic eczema are geared toward lowering the number of circulating IgE antibodies, and lowering cutaneous cytokines, chemokines, activated mast cell, and Th2 T-cells which promote inflammation.[3,4] However, standard treatment, usually in the form of topical steroids, leaves many gaps because they only treat part of the problem.

The healthy immune system is balanced between two components: Th1, geared to innate immunity, addresses infections, such as colds and unfamiliar novel antigens. And Th2, acquired immunity, which houses the memory that mobilizes in response to antigens we have encountered before. Normally, Th1 will be dominant, as we will likely encounter many unfamiliar minor antigens. It is the active controller of the immune system, which will alert the Th2 system when reinforcements will be needed, as for a virulent infection, or a complex organism like a parasite. Healthy skin plays a crucial role in this. It can respond to a local breach such as a cut or scrape and isolate the rest of the body from any wider infection.

One of the many jobs of the Th2 immune system is to make IgE immunoglobulins (antibody); IgE antibodies initiate the allergic response when they intercept a specific trigger (like dust, pollen, specific foods, etc). In the presence of that trigger (antigen), IgE antibodies will bind to receptors on mast cells and activate the allergic response. Activated mast cells will dump massive amounts of histamine and other mediators into the blood stream, which together cause the flushing, itching, swelling, and catastrophic drops in blood pressure we see in allergic reactions. This mechanism underlies acute and chronic allergic conditions, where genetically susceptible individuals produce antigen-specific IgE antibodies to harmless environmental triggers, and initiate unnecessary inflammatory reactions.

To visualize the healthy immune balance, think of it as a seesaw with a parent and a child. One end of the seesaw is always up in the air and the other is always on the ground. The parent can make a game of it by pushing up with their legs, but "normal" is when the child is stuck up in the air.

In the case of a chronic disease, such as eczema, the body is never normal. Th1 is too weak, and Th2 is too strong. Patients may try over-the-counter antihistamines to reverse the downstream histamine release caused by overactive Th2, but there is little evidence to support or refute its efficacy as monotherapy for eczema. Topical corticosteroids (TCS), which suppress both Th1 and Th2, are the first-line treatment for eczema but they are strong, and the side effect profile is significant; for example, TCS used consistently for only one month causes skin barrier fragility and will actually worsen eczematic lesions, and importantly, more potent TCS formulations can cause transient depression of the adrenal glands, which produce hormones that drive growth and development in children. Further, up to 30% of patients will have eczema that does not respond to TCS, and one in ten of those patients will go on to require systemic corticosteroid therapy. Systemic corticosteroids cannot be used long term because they significantly alter the body's biochemistry and cause more harm than good; they can even cause a *paradoxical increase in IgE* — *and* remember, too much IgE caused the symptoms in the first place! Corticosteroids provide relief by suppressing the Th2 response, but they also suppress Th1, which leaves the body more vulnerable to other infections and other significant side effects.

After steroids are discontinued, the imbalance remains. Think of the seesaw: the child has suddenly grown up. B cells are more activated. IgE and eosinophils are rampant and damage the tissue that is supposed to protect against infection. Skin dries out, leading to infection and the oozing described by many patients. This state of immune imbalance is sometimes referred to as inflammation/Th2 rebound, i.e., worse than before steroid use. In this stage, there is further elevation of IgE and eosinophilic inflammation circulating in the blood. It also called "hyper serum IgE", which is really shorthand for an overabundance of a toxic stew of inflammatory agents released by a cycle of inappropriate immune responses. "Hyper serum IgE" is different from "Hyper IgE syndrome", which is a genetic disorder.

The quest for relief encourages a pattern of use and relapse and may foster a lifestyle of habitual topical corticosteroid use, which has a slew of negative side effects, but can also lead to medication tolerance, and then in extreme cases, medication addiction — where the skin requires longer courses and more frequent topical corticosteroid therapy in order to achieve a therapeutic response. In the meantime, reduced innate immunity leaves the patient vulnerable to opportunistic infection that would normally be dealt with via Th1 mechanisms.

Signs of corticosteroid addiction are variable. Pediatric patients with addicted skin may first subjectively notice that application of topical corticosteroids no longer provides the same relief. Some patients notice no improvement of the eczematous lesions at all. Some patients develop worsening pruritis and skin lesions at the beginning of topical steroid therapy which persist as intractable nodules, or prurigo, upon completion of the steroid regimen.[5]

Patients with topical corticosteroid withdrawal may experience mild rebound eruption consisting of flushing or erythema with or without edema. Most patients will experience intractable eczema and erythema where they had applied topical steroid cream and notice that day by day, they continue to spread.[5] It will eventually affect areas where topical corticosteroids were never applied, and often follows a pattern of rebound eruption starting at the face, then spreading down to the neck, upper extremities, trunk, and then lower extremities. In severe cases, patients may experience papules, pustules, or skin erosions, which may or may not be accompanied by fever. After the acute phase, the skin thickens, callouses and then desquamates, which is immensely uncomfortable in raw, eczematous skin. Secondary infection with skin-inhabiting microbes (*S. aureus, S. epidermidus*) is of great concern due to the expansiveness of desquamated (broken) skin, and the weakened Th1 response. The course of rebound eruption may last a few days or a few months, and to date there are no FDA-approved therapies to control the symptoms.

Filling the Gaps with TCM

Traditional Chinese medicine (TCM) has broad therapeutic effects. The same combination of herbs and their constituents may possess anti-inflammatory, antimicrobial, antifungal, and other therapeutic values simultaneously.[6,7] That is, they may fight active infection at the same time they are calming inflammation and repairing the barrier function and long-term integrity of the skin. A later pharmacology study revealed many of the immune elements of this therapy are relevant to the restoration of T cell and B cells and innate immune regulation,[8,9] and skin barrier/integrity such as vitamin D receptors, and PPAR γ, which contribute to skin healing.[10]

Evidence of Relief Through Traditional Chinese Medicine: A Case of a 7-Year-Old Male

While there are no FDA-approved treatments for severe refractory atopic eczema characterized by corticosteroid addiction and withdrawal, patients have experienced transformative results using TCM. Consider this published case of a 7-year-old male with allergic eczema since the age of 2 months who presented with persistent, refractory atopic dermatitis despite chronic mid-potency topical corticosteroid use and an 18-month trial of step-up therapy to high-potency topical corticosteroids. He was diagnosed with steroid with-drawal syndrome with the complication of *Staphylococcus aureus* infection confirmed by skin culture. He responded poorly to antibiotics (oral cephalexin and topical mupirocin) combined with pulse steroid therapy by injection.

The patient received multicomponent TCM therapy of herbal bath addi-tive, herbal creams, and internal teas. Within one week of treatment, his lesions showed signs of improvement. By 1 month of treatment, the inten-sity of his skin lesions improved; oozing, erythema, and excoriation resolved. His SCORAD values decreased by 79% (from 103 to 21.8) after 1 month of TCM and by 99% following 3–6 months of TCM. Notably, throughout TCM treatment he did not require use of oral or topical steroids. His total serum IgE decreased 75% (from 19,000 kIU/L to 4,630 kIU/L) by 12 months (see Table 12.1). Absolute eosinophil counts decreased by 60% (from 1×103 to 0.427×103 cells/μL). His skin remained well controlled while on mainte-nance of TCM regimen, and by 17 months of treatment he was able to taper and discontinue the regimen without any flare-up. His skin continued to be well controlled at least 3 months after discontinuation of TCM.

The Transformative Response of TCM: Proposed Mechanism

The mechanism of action is likely due to multiple TCM components that target the IgE-mediated eczema pathway. In vitro studies have shown that the herbal internal tea used for this patient has anti-IgE, eotaxin and TNF-α effects. Previous studies showed the herbal tea component has empirically inhibited Th2 cytokine IL-4 production, which mediates IgE production.[8] *Radix glycyrrhizae*, a specific herbal component, has been shown to inhibit LPS induced NF-$\varkappa$B activation, a key player in eczema disease pathogene-sis,[11] and its compound 7,4 dihydroxyflavone inhibits Th2-mediated cytokine production.[12] *Flos lonicerae* has antibacterial action against skin microbes such as *Staphlococcus aureus* and streptocococci, and exhibits an anti-inflammatory and hepatic cell protective effect.[13]

References

1. Odhiambo JA, *et al.* Global variations in prevalence of eczema symptoms in children from ISAAC Phase Three. *J Allergy Clin Immunol.* 2009;124(6):1251–8e23.
2. Proudfoot LE, *et al.* The European TREatment of severe Atopic eczema in children Taskforce (TREAT) survey. *Br J Dermatol.* 2013;169(4): 901–909.
3. Ng C, *et al.* Hyper IgE in childhood eczema and risk of asthma in Chinese children. *Molecules.* 2016 Jun 10;21(6):753.
4. Lewis-Jones S, Mugglestone MA, G. Guideline Development. Management of atopic eczema in children aged up to 12 years: summary of NICE guidance. *BMJ.* 2007;335(7632):1263–1264.
5. Fukaya M. Histological and immunohistological findings using anti-cortisol antibody in atopic dermatitis with topical steroid addiction. *Dermatol Ther (Heidelb).* 2016;6(1):39–46.
6. Wang Z, *et al.* Traditional Chinese medicine for food allergy and eczema. *Ann Allergy Asthma Immunol.* 2021 Jun;126(6):639–654.
7. Lisann L, *et al.* Successful prevention of extremely frequent and severe food anaphylaxis in three children by combined traditional Chinese medicine therapy. *Allergy Asthma Clin Immunol.* 2014;10(1):66.
8. Thanik E, *et al.* Effect of traditional Chinese medicine on skin lesions and quality of life in patients with moderate to severe eczema. *Ann Allergy Asthma Immunol.* 2018;121(1):135–136.
9. Srivastava K, *et al.* Effect of Traditional Chinese Medicine (TCM) in moderate-to-severe eczema in clinic and animal model: beyond corticosteroids. *J Allergy Clin Immunol.* 2020;145(2):AB198.
10. Wang ZZ, *et al.* Systems pharmacology and in silico docking analysis uncover association of CA2, PPARG, RXRA, and VDR with the mechanisms underlying the Shi Zhen Tea formula effect on eczema. *Evid Based Complement Alternat Med.* 2021;2021:8406127.
11. Thanik E, *et al.* Improvement of skin lesions and life quality in moderate-to-severe eczema patients by combined TCM therapy. *Ann Allergy Asthma Immunol.* 2018;12(1).
12. Kim YW, *et al.* Anti-inflammatory effects of liquiritigenin as a consequence of the inhibition of NF-kappaB-dependent iNOS and proinflammatory cytokines production. *Br J Pharmacol.* 2008;154(1):165–173.

12. Yang N, *et al.* Glycyrrhiza uralensis flavonoids present in anti-asthma formula, ASHMI™, inhibit memory Th2 responses in vitro and in vivo. *Phytother Res.* 2013;27(9):1381–1391.

13. Huang K. Antibacterial, antiviral, and anti-fungal herbs. In: *The Pharmacology of Chinese Herbs.* CRC Press, Boca Raton, London New York, Washington, D.C., 1999, Chap. 36, pp. 388–389.

ECZEMA, FOOD ALLERGY, AND TRADITIONAL CHINESE MEDICINE (TCM) THERAPY

Johnathan Neshiwat, Medical Student, Researcher*
and Xiu-Min Li, MD, MS[†]

*Lake Erie College of Osteopathic Medicine, Erie, Pennsylvania 16509, USA
[†]New York Medical College, Valhalla, New York 10595, USA

Abstract

The prevalence of food allergy has been steadily increasing. It has an estimated impact of $24.8 billion on the economy affecting 2.0% to 5.0% of children. Eczema affects an estimated 20% of children with an economic burden of $5.37 billion. Food allergy currently has no multi-food tolerance treatment. Eczema is typically treated with topical corticosteroids. Corticosteroids are not suitable for long-term use because they can become refractory. Eczema can have serious complications such as infection, lymphoma, pruritus, and even non-melanoma skin cancer. Traditional Chinese medicine (TCM) has been introduced in the healthcare setting as an effective treatment for both food allergy and eczema. Independent treatment of food allergy using TCM has shown successful reversal of food intolerance. Systematic review of eczema treatment using TCM has demonstrated improvement of health-related quality of life in children with moderate-to-severe disease.

Keywords: Food allergy, topical corticosteroids, eczema, non-melanoma skin cancer

Food Allergy and TCM Therapy

It is thought that the prevalence of food allergy in the United States has been steadily increasing[1] with the highest prevalence in children.[1] The expected prevalence of peanut allergy among schoolchildren ranges from 2.0% to 5.0% of the United States population, dependent on definition.[2] Food allergy poses a serious financial concern for the average family, costing an estimated $4184 per child or $24.8 billion on the economy.[3] The FDA has approved a peanut-specific treatment for food intolerance, Palforzia. However, there are no current treatments for multiple food allergen tolerance aside from avoidance. For these children, there is serious concern of decreased growth trajectory and nutritional status.[4*] Treatment of food allergy can be measured by two metrics: desensitization and tolerance. Desensitization is characterized by an allergic reaction that is mitigated by medication. Tolerance refers to treatment that diminishes the immunologic response to the food allergen.[5] Long-term immunologic reactions to food allergens are precipitated by an IgE memory response.[6]

TCM Therapy for Reversal of Food Intolerance

TCM has been utilized as a mainstream method of reducing IgE production due to its potent anti-inflammatory properties. TCM has proven effective reversal of food intolerance in a child who had lost 49 foods and gained none. Two years after TCM therapy, 35 foods were introduced, and no additional foods were lost. The patient was able to decrease the number of foods avoided by 43%, reintroducing 21 of the previously avoided foods (Fig. 11.1a and Fig. 11.1b). Prior to TCM therapy, the patient had downtrending IgE in 3 foods, which increased to 12 after TCM therapy was

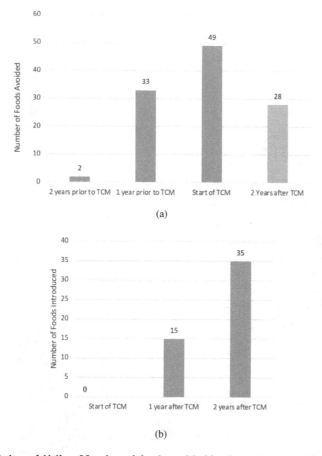

Figures 11. 1a and 11.1b.   Number of foods avoided by the patient, stratified by time. The patient continued to lose food tolerance until the start of the TCM when they were successfully able to introduce 35 foods.

initiated. Additionally, the patient had up-trending IgE caused by 9 foods which was reduced to 5 after TCM (Fig. 11.2).[4]

Food-specific IgE was measured for 12 different foods at numerous occasions prior to TCM and the trends for IgE readings were noted. Prior to TCM, most foods showed a trend of steadily increasing readings of food-specific IgE. Very few foods were down-trending over numerous readings of food-specific IgE prior to TCM. After TCM, food-specific IgE was measured

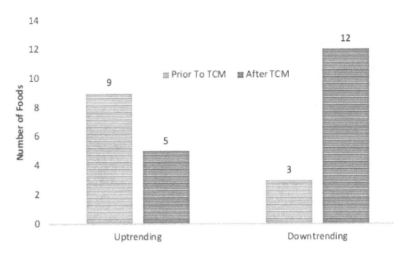

Figure 11.2. Trends in food-specific IgE over multiple lab tests before and after TCM.

numerous times for the same 12 foods, plus 3 additional foods. Fortunately, after TCM, most foods showed a drastic shift in trend, where the majority were now down-trending in food-specific IgE. Only five foods were up-trending over numerous readings of food-specific IgE after TCM.

Eczema and TCM Therapy

Eczema is a chronic-relapsing dermatologic inflammatory condition affecting 1 in 5 children and impacting quality of life.[7] 91% of atopic dermatitis patients have flare-up symptoms on a daily basis and 75% have sought medical attention for their condition.[7] Additionally, increased risks of infection, lymphoma, pruritus, and non-melanoma skin cancer have also been reported in eczema patients.[9] It places a financial burden of $5.37 billion on the United States economy.[7] Theories surrounding the pathogenesis of eczema are focused on the weakened skin barrier that allows for allergen exposure.[8] This could either be caused by inflammation allowing allergens to penetrate the immune system (as per the inside-out hypothesis) or a weakened skin barrier that causes allergen exposure and immune dysregulation (as per the outside-in hypothesis).[8]

Eczema prevalence and impact on quality of life are serious concerns. Current mainstay therapy includes corticosteroids, which can become refractory to treatment and have serious adverse reactions.[10] Paradoxically, corticosteroids can even cause dermatologic inflammation.[10] Therefore, a more reliable long-term alternative to steroids is necessary. The use of TCM therapy in patients with eczema has been well studied. Independent systematic review of publications from 2013–2016 had found an improvement of health-related quality of life in children with moderate to severe disease.[11] TCM has been shown to treat corticosteroid-associated eczema itching, skin lesions, and even associated sleep disturbances.[10] TCM Therapy has been shown to be well tolerated.[10]

References

1. Tang ML, Mullins RJ. Food allergy: is prevalence increasing? *Intern Med J.* 2017;47(3):256–261. doi:10.1111/imj.13362
2. Bunyavanich S, Rifas-Shiman SL, Platts-Mills TA, *et al.* Peanut allergy prevalence among school-age children in a US cohort not selected for any disease. *J Allergy Clin Immunol.* 2014;134(3):753–755. doi:10.1016/j.jaci.2014.05.050
3. Gupta R, Holdford D, Bilaver L, Dyer A, Holl JL, Meltzer D. The economic impact of childhood food allergy in the United States. *JAMA Pediatr.* 2013;167(11):1026–1031.
4. Soffer G, Neshiwat J, McKnight T, Park S, Chung D, Li XM. Successful reversal of multiple food sensitivities/intolerances with Traditional Chinese Medicine in a pediatric patient. Submitted 2021.
5. Tang ML, Mullins RJ. Food allergy: is prevalence increasing? *Intern Med J.* 2017;47(3):256–261. doi:10.1111/imj.13362
6. Moutsoglou DM, Dreskin SC. B cells establish, but do not maintain, long-lived murine anti-peanut IgE(a). *Clin Exp Allergy.* 2016;46(4):640–653. doi:10.1111/cea.12715
7. Avena-Woods C. Overview of atopic dermatitis. *Am J Manag Care.* 2017;23(8 Suppl):S115–S123.
8. Silverberg NB, Silverberg JI. Inside out or outside in: does atopic dermatitis disrupt barrier function or does disruption of barrier function trigger atopic dermatitis? *Cutis.* 2015;96(6):359–361.

9. Eichenfield LF, Tom WL, Berger TG, Krol A, Paller AS, Schwarzenberger K, Bergman JN, Chamlin SL, Cohen DE, Cooper KD, Cordoro KM, Davis DM, Feldman SR, Hanifin JM, Margolis DJ, Silverman RA, Simpson EL, Williams HC, Elmets CA, Block J, Harrod CG, Smith Begolka W, Sidbury R. Guidelines of care for the management of atopic dermatitis: ection 2. Management and treatment of atopic dermatitis with topical therapies. *J Am Acad Dermatol.* 2014;71(1):116–132.

10. Wang Z, Wang ZZ, Geliebter J, Tiwari R, Li XM. Traditional Chinese medicine for food allergy and eczema. *Ann Allergy Asthma Immunol.* 2021 Jun;126(6):639–654.

11. Gu SX, Zhang AL, Coyle ME, Chen D, Xue CC. Chinese herbal medicine for atopic eczema: an overview of clinical evidence. *J Dermatol Treat.* 2017;28(3):246–250. doi:10.1080/09546634.2016.1214673

Part II
Patients and Their Stories

Dr. Xiu-Min Li has treated hundreds of patients successfully for recalcitrant eczema as well as a range of co-morbid immune and autoimmune disorders. Chapter 12 provides detailed clinical notes on three of those patients, as well as her ideas on disease and treatment classification. Chapters 13–36 are 24 cases told from the point of view of patients and family members. Stories have been shared with the permission of patients and parents, although names have been changed, and in one case, facial photographs are used with the written permission of the subject, age 12, as well as his mother. Our friend Dr. Renata Engler has observed of her colleagues, "We have lost connection with patient stories. Patients who don't fit are marginalized. Doctors should expand their medical toolbox for patients who don't fall within guidelines." These are stories of patients who have connected with a treating physician who expanded the toolbox and brought them back from the margins.

All patients were treated at
INTEGRATIVE HEALTH & ACUPUNCTURE, PC.
933 Mamaroneck Ave, Mamaroneck, NY 10543

BEYOND CORTICOSTEROIDS: STRATEGIES AND MILESTONES OF THE HEALING PROCESS

Xiu-Min Li, MD, MS

Department of Pathology, Microbiology and Immunology,
and Department of Otolaryngology
New York Medical College, Valhalla, New York 10595, USA

Introduction

Eczema is a chronic inflammatory skin condition. Topical corticosteroids are first-line treatment and generally effective. However, some patients become steroid refractory, requiring progressively higher-potency doses, and sometimes one or more courses of systemic steroids.[1] Long-term topical steroid use may lead to dependence even as effectiveness declines. Prompted by concern over adverse effects from chronic steroid use as well as diminishing effectiveness, individuals may undergo steroid withdrawal (also called red skin syndrome). During this period, skin lesions will worsen.

Eczema in children is often associated with allergies, such as food allergy, asthma, and environmental allergies, which further complicate treatment. In young children, frequent flares and multiple food sensitivity may delay food introduction. Therefore, therapy that accounts for the whole person, not just the skin, would be a new vision of health care and fulfill the criteria set by NIH/National Center for Complementary and Integrative Health Strategies. We developed a unique TCM therapy based on traditional Chinese medicine (TCM) practice, research, our understanding of pathological mechanisms of eczema and food allergy, and other inflammatory conditions. It has shown efficacy in treating eczema patients, including young children, improved severity scores, reduced pruritus, and lowered corticosteroid use, resulting in better quality of life, with no serious adverse effects. It also showed beneficial immunological effects on IgE, Th2, and inflammatory cytokines. We also began to identify active compounds and therapeutic targets using computational modeling, in vitro and in vivo models.[2,3] This chapter will present strategies and milestones of healing process for recalcitrance, steroid-dependency, or steroid withdrawal associated with severe eczema along with strategies of early introduction of TCM for young infants with acute eczema, and discuss our current clinical and laboratory research.

New View of Eczema Types and Case Presentation

Eczema is a syndrome that represents a group of skin inflammatory symptoms. Eczema can be categorized into 4 types based on age, clinical skin eczema severity, and steroid use status.

Type I. Infant and Young Children with Steroid-Dependent/Recalcitrant Eczema

This type of eczema covers infant and young children ages 6 months to 4 years. They have been on steroids for at least 3 months with multiple unsuccessful attempts to stop. Eczema would typically return within days or weeks of discontinuing the medication, requiring reintroduction, or sometimes, use of oral steroids. For a while, their skin will be adequately controlled. However, over time this responsive phase will fade and progress to steroid recalcitrance. The term "steroid recalcitrant" means "difficult to treat". In this stage, the skin is still afflicted while on the topical medication, and much worse when its use is halted. This is also a stage when young children tend to develop multiple-food sensitization, or intolerance. It is worth noting that this status of steroid dependent/recalcitrant is one of the major risk factors that make individuals most vulnerable to developing steroid withdrawal syndrome (See Type III eczema below). Therefore, with Type I, when infant and young children with steroid-dependent and recalcitrant eczema commence TCM therapy, the general advice is that they continue their established steroid protocol provided by their dermatologist, allergist, pediatrician, or other health providers, along with dietary supplements, to prevent sudden steroid withdrawal issues. The TCM multi-component therapy is a clinically well-established protocol named "triple TCM therapy". It contains internal herbal tea, herbal baths, and external herbal creams. These children respond to triple TCM therapy relatively quickly. Compliance levels are excellent because parents, who have watched their children suffer, are committed to the protocol. The case series study published by *Annals of Allergy, Asthma and Immunology* in 2021[4] and included in Chapter 3 of this book, showed that within one month of treatment, skin lesions improve by 80–100% at 3 months of treatment with 90–100% improvement at 6 months of treatment. During 1–3 months of triple TCM therapy, steroid use is substantially reduced, but caution is needed about dropping their usage too fast. Therefore, triple TCM therapy plays a complementary role at the beginning to help individuals taper steroids. As treatment progresses, triple TCM therapy plays a key role in continuing skin healing.

Type II. Older Children and Young Adults with Steroid-Dependent Severe Eczema

These patients have many more cases of chronic eczema than other groups. Also, due to the process known as the "atopic march", many of them have already developed other allergies including environmental allergy and food allergy. Sometimes, their multiple allergic conditions started in young childhood, generally with eczema as the first. These children also face more social challenges since they are attending school with attendant social issues on top of medical ones. Itching/painful, unsightly skin lesions and loss of sleep lead to a very stressful life. Nevertheless, the triple therapy helps if the individual can commit to the protocol. The healing process is generally slower than with Type I eczema. The successful cases are presented in our recent publications — Fig. 2 by Wang *et al.*[4] and by Thanik *et al.*[5] — and an additional case below.

An 18-year-old female visited Integrative Health and Acupuncture PC, Mamaroneck, NY from Canada with her family right before the pandemic in February 2020 for her severe eczema. This patient has had pediatrician-diagnosed eczema since she was 2 months old and had been on nearly daily topical treatment with Aveeno, Desitin, or hydrocortisone. Her eczema was manageable until June 2019 when her skin lesions became so severe. She had been seen by a dermatologist who had recommended oral steroid or Dupixent (the biologic *dupilumab*). At the first office visit, her entire body was covered with all stages of eczema lesion including erythema, edema/papulation, crust, excoriation, lichenification, and dryness; lichenification and dryness are the most extreme (Fig. 12.1(a) and Fig. 12.2(a)).

Upon her return home, she started triple TCM therapy. At the first month or 2 her skin condition continued to deteriorate, and she was exceedingly fatigued, unable to walk, and had daytime somnolence related to restless sleep during the night. Her menstrual cycle also stopped. This was at the beginning of the pandemic, when herbal supplies were erratic. An ER dermatologist and her primary physician put her on 2 courses of oral prednisone, which helped slightly. Dr. Li conducted phone consultations every

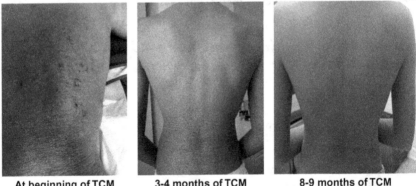

| At beginning of TCM | 3-4 months of TCM | 8-9 months of TCM |
| (a) | (b) | (c) |

Figure 12.1. Improvement of skin on the back with TCM. (a) Skin on the back at beginning of TCM showing excoriation, lichenification, redness, dryness. (b) 3–4 months of TCM showing mild to moderate improvement. (c) 8–9 months of TCM showing remarkable improvement.

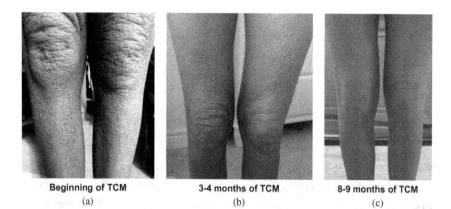

| Beginning of TCM | 3-4 months of TCM | 8-9 months of TCM |
| (a) | (b) | (c) |

Figure 12.2. Improvement of leg skin lesions with TCM. (a) Front of legs showing severe lichenification on knees, many cuts at the front legs at the beginning of TCM. (b) 3–4 months of TCM showing slight improvement. (c) 8–9 months of TCM showing marked improvement. The blue color is from the herbal external cream.

2–4 weeks to work with the family on supporting the protocol. There were no obvious side effects from ceasing oral steroids. By 3–4 months (June 2020), her skin started to stabilize and show signs of improvement (Fig. 12.1(b) and Fig. 12.2(b)). The turning point came at 8–9 months of triple TCM therapy. Her skin improved by up to 90% and many parts of her body looked normal. Her skin had no open scabs or wounds. (Fig. 12.1(c) and Fig. 12.2(c)). Her menstrual cycle returned, and she started to regain lost weight, return to college classes, and take music lessons. Her immunological markers were also showing signs of improvement, such as absolute eosinophils dropping from 2.2 to 0.9 (normal range $0{\sim}0.7 \times 10^3$ cells/μL). Total IgE fell from 19,000 μg/L (equal to 7977 ku/L) to 4,765 ku/L and liver and kidney function test results were all in the normal range. Her skin scores have been monitored using the standard SCORAD and have reduced from 102.66 to 5.18 (over 95% reduction). Her skin continued to improve. By nearly the 1-year mark, she completed phase I milestone of TCM therapy and moved to phase II and early phase III protocol. The dose and frequency of her herbal protocol were reduced.

In summary, this case presents a unique characteristic of eczema for chronicity, severity, and type of disease. The patient has achieved her initial goal of reducing unsightly lesions, reducing itching, and sleep improvement. However, it took her longer than is typical for completing the phase I protocol. The new goal is to continue to build skin integrity and strengthen its barrier function, which will allow her to further reduce triple therapy protocol and to stop daily treatment. This is equally important as phase I protocol.

Type III. Red Skin Syndrome/Steroid Addiction/ Steroid Withdrawal Syndrome

Steroid dependence (abuse) or steroid withdrawal result in sleep disturbance, extreme redness/oozing/crust/pealing, itching, painful skin, and stress, which are mediated by complex inflammatory cell and cytokine networks and altered skin integrity. It used to be believed that this type of situation occurs only in adults, but we now see it in children. The treatment options are extremely limited. Patients would suffer from these conditions for years, severely limiting the quality of life of patients and their families. Our previously published case series showed that triple TCM therapy has steroid-sparing effects and holds great promise to improve skin lesions and quality of life.[5] The following represent different ages.

Case 1

A 45-year-old female with eczema since she was a child and diagnosed by a pediatrician. Throughout her adulthood, she had been struggling with her eczema. She had been through steroids, light treatment, and many prescription solutions including the expensive biologic Dupixent, which she started in April 2017 and stopped in December 2019. She stopped because her hair started to fall out, and because she displayed extreme facial redness. She said it looked like a fungal infection. Three months after stopping Dupixent, her skin was manageable, but she started to show red skin syndrome. She started light treatment with a dermatologist in October 2019 until COVID-19 started around March 2020, which resulted in some improvement, although her skin was still very symptomatic. The dermatologist wanted to give her a stronger steroid or methotrexate, a potent immune-suppressing drug also used for cancer, but she refused. She started multi-component TCM therapy through Integrative Health and Acupuncture PC, Mamaroneck, NY in June 2020. Since it was in the middle of the pandemic, in-person visits were not possible. The patient provided comprehensive medical history information, skin photos, and copy of laboratory test data ordered by her primary physicians prior to the consultation. At the first consult, she showed severe lesions on her face, neck, upper chest, back, arms, and hands. She was exceedingly itchy and slept poorly (both scored 10 on the 0–10 scale) for many months. Her moods were mercurial, and she had severe fatigue (Score 3 on the 0–3 scale). Medications included antihistamines cetirizine and the sedating hydroxyzine, which, along with the tranquilizer diazepam (Valium), was taken for sleep. She also had physician-diagnosed environmental allergies. Her laboratory test showed that her total IgE was exceedingly high, >10,000kU/L (normal <200 kIU/L). She also developed more food and environmental allergen IgE sensitization over the years (not shown) and high eosinophil accounts (0.53×10^3 cells/μL, normal range 0–0.3×10^3 cells/μL) and high % of eosinophils (9.4%, normal range 0–6%). She mentioned that she had never had such high total IgE and specific IgEs against so many food and environmental allergens.

She started triple TCM therapy including internal tea, external bath, and external cream as published in Chapter 3 of this book. After 3 months, her skin lesions were markedly improved. There were no crusts, scabs, open wounds, etc. Sleeping and itching score were reduced from 10 to 0. Fig. 12.3(a) shows hands before TCM and Fig. 12.3(b) shows hands after

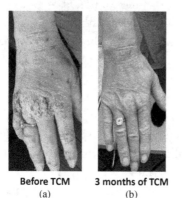

Before TCM   3 months of TCM
(a)   (b)

Figure 12.3. Improvement of eczema lesion. (a) Prior to TCM, showing all stages of lesion including erythema, edema, crust, excoriation, lichenification, and dryness. (b) 3 months of TCM, showing improvement in erythema, edema, crust, and excoriation, and skin is in the healing process.

3 months of TCM. Her arms, chest, and back were nearly normal, her hands were dry, and her face was still red sometimes in response to irritation such as heat. At 6 months of TCM her SCORAD reduced from 95 (before TCM) to 1.4 (over 95% improvement). She completed phase I and phase II protocols to further stabilize her skin. At approximately month-6 lab follow up, her total IgE reduced to 7610 IU/L and eosinophil count and % were all in the normal range (2.6% and 0.13×10^3 cell/L respectively).

In summary, this patient had gone through substantial topical steroids, light therapy, and biological drug treatment. Her skin lesions were at a severe stage and her quality of life was badly affected prior to seeking TCM therapy. Triple TCM therapy improved her skin lesions and quality of life in 3 months without adverse steroidal effects. As an adult who suffered from chronic eczema, the improvement on her skin and the whole person is important. The plan for continuation is to increase skin integrity and build a stronger platform with TCM so that her skin will be able to adapt to changing environments without triggering her condition.

Case 2

A 7-year-old male with atopic dermatitis from 2 months of age had presented with persistent refractory eczema despite chronic mid-potency topical corticosteroid use and an 18-month trial of step-up therapy to high-potency topical corticosteroids. Over a 6-month period prior to TCM, he had used 8 courses of prednisolone. However, the eczematous lesions returned as soon as 3 days after completing the last course of prednisolone and progressed to total body erythroderma over 12 days, with increased severity compared to that prior to using the systemic steroid. He was diagnosed with steroid withdrawal syndrome with the complication of *Staphylococcus aureus* infection confirmed by skin culture. He responded poorly to antibiotics (oral cephalexin and topical mupirocin) combined with injection of steroids. His primary allergist referred him to receive TCM therapy from Dr. Li, who referred him to a secondary allergist and a dermatologist for evaluation before starting TCM therapy at the Integrative Health and Acupuncture PC in New York.

Upon the first visit for TCM therapy in June 2016, the patient presented with total body erythroderma characterized further by severe erythema,

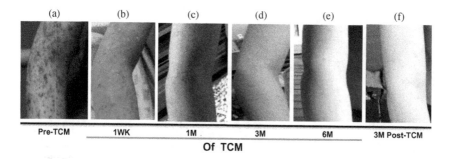

(a)	(b)	(c)	(d)	(e)	(f)
Pre-TCM	1WK	1M	3M	6M	3M Post-TCM

Of TCM

Figure 12.4. Improvement of skin lesions during TCM therapy. (a) Prior to TCM, showing severe skin lesions. (b–e) Showing improvement during TCM therapy (internal tea, external herbal bath and cream). Skin started to improve in 1 week, continued to improve, and nearly completely improved in 6 months. No steroids or antibiotics were used during the course of TCM therapy.

edema, oozing, and excoriations as well as extensive blistering and bleeding (Fig. 12.4(a)). Disease was deemed severe based on a score of 103 by standardized SCORAD. He was unable to walk secondary to pain and had daytime somnolence related to restless sleep during the night. His medical history was significant for multiple food allergies and allergic rhinitis associated with perennial and seasonal allergen sensitization. He reported uncontrollable pruritus despite taking cetirizine once daily, oral hydroxyzine HCL (Atarax) every six hours, and diphenhydramine as needed. Laboratory results provided by his primary allergist indicated elevated total serum IgE (19,000 kIU/L, normal 100kIU/L), eosinophilia (1×10^3 cells/μL, normal range 0–0.3×10^3 cells/μL) (Table 12.1), and high specific IgE levels to multiple food and environmental allergens (not shown). He had positive allergen skin tests to peanut, egg, and cat in 2015. He had a history of anaphylaxis from peanuts, eggs, milk, and seeds, despite a negative milk skin test. Egg caused wheezing, while milk, peanut, soy, and wheat caused rash. His aspartate aminotransferase, alanine transaminase, and blood urea nitrogen levels were all within normal range.

The patient received triple TCM therapy of herbal bath additive, herbal creams, and internal teas, described previously.[5] Within one week of treatment, his lesions showed signs of improvement (Fig. 12.4(b)). By 1 month of treatment, his skin lesions intensity was significantly improved; there was no oozing, erythema, or excoriation, but with persistence of dryness and

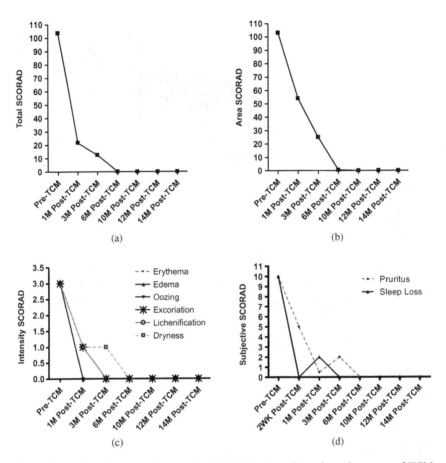

Figure 12.5. Scoring Atopic Dermatitis (SCORAD) values throughout the course of TCM treatment. (A) Total overall SCORAD values. (B) SCORAD values of regional areas affected by dermatitis. (C) SCORAD values indicating objective findings of dermatitis intensity. (D) SCORAD values indicating subjective findings of pruritus and quality of sleep.

lichenification (Fig. 12.4(c)). His SCORAD values decreased by 79% (from 103 to 21.8) after 1 month of TCM and by 99% following 3–6 months of TCM (Fig. 12.4(d)–Fig. 12.4(e), Fig. 12.5).

Most strikingly, he showed rapid improvement in sleep quality within one week and the patient reported no itching by two weeks of treatment. Notably, throughout TCM treatment, he did not require use of oral or topical steroids.

Table 12.1. Improvement of laboratory immunological measures and inflammation.

	PRE-TCM	12M of TCM	Reference Range
Total Serum IgE (K/uL)	19,000	4,630	<100
WBC (cells/uL)	11	6.1	4.3–12.4
Hemoglobin (g/dL)	13.7	13.1	10.9–14.8
Platelets (K/uL)	479	382	190–459
Absolute Eosinophil (×10³)	1	0.4	0–0.3
Creatinine (mg/dL)	0.54	0.48	0.37–0.62
Aspartate Aminotransferase (U/L)	29	26	0–60
Alanine Aminotransferase (U/L)	20	12	0–25

His total serum IgE decreased 75% (from 19,000 kIU/L to 4,630 kIU/L) by 12 months (Table 12.1). Absolute eosinophil counts decreased by 60% (from 1×10^3 to 0.427×10^3 cells/μL). Liver and kidney function tests remained within normal range (Table 1). His skin remained well controlled while on maintenance of TCM regimen, and by 17 months of TCM he was able to taper and discontinue the TCM regimen without any flare-up. His skin continued to be well controlled at least 3 months after the discontinuation of TCM (Fig. 12.4(f)). He even experienced improvement of documented anaphylactic food allergies, including reintroduction of wheat and soy at 6 months post TCM, and successfully passing a milk challenge in 2019, one year after completing TCM therapy.

In summary, we present a case of steroid withdrawal syndrome treated with multicomponent TCM in a 7-year-old child with chronic eczema since infancy. In our case, his allergist, dermatologist, and the local Children's hospital emergency care physicians ruled out hyper IgE syndrome, a genetic disorder with STAT3 mutation, because the patient did not have characteristic facial and dental abnormalities or recurrent lung infections associated with this syndrome.[6,7] Instead, it is believed that the isolated hyper serum IgE seen on laboratory studies was due to his chronic and severe eczema and overuse of steroids, or steroid withdrawal. As supportive evidence, his IgE was markedly reduced after TCM therapy at the 1-year mark when his skin lesions have markedly improved, whereas syndromic hyper IgE would not resolve with therapy.

Case 3

A 34-month-old female with eczema for 2 years, including steroid withdrawal for 1 year. Medical history was provided by parents. She started to have eczema when she was 5 months, diagnosed by a pediatrician. Family tried 1% hydrocortisone OTC, but did not show improvement, and she had an infection. It started on the face and spread to the whole body. She was treated with mometasone and antibiotics. It was working initially for a year, as more than 50% of the time she was on mometasone. When she was 24 months old, a dermatologist suggested triamcinolone, but the family did not use it. The family was concerned about the cycle. After reading extensively, her parents decided not to continue with topical steroids. In February 2020, they stopped all topical steroids. Her skin progressively worsened over 6 months. It was the most severe 2 weeks prior to initial consultation.

During steroid withdrawal, she used Mupirocin 3 times because the skin was oozing. The last use of Mupirocin was also two weeks before the TCM consult. First consult, virtually, at Integrative Health and Acupuncture PC was in April 2021. Her face, neck, back of the knee, behind the ears, and inner elbow are most severe, showing oozing, crust, redness, excoriation, and edema. The face lesions are shown in Fig. 12.6(a). She had severe pruritus score 10 on the 0–10 scale and poor sleep (score of 10 on the 0–10 scale). She awakened up to 6 times a night. Her SCORAD was 92.3.

The family's goal in seeking TCM therapy is to treat eczema and steroid withdrawal, no more oozing, improve sleep, and reducing itching. She started

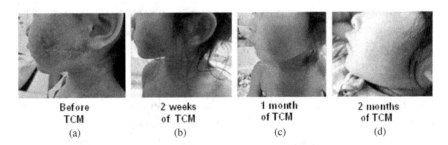

| Before TCM | 2 weeks of TCM | 1 month of TCM | 2 months of TCM |
| (a) | (b) | (c) | (d) |

Figure 12.6. Improved skin lesions on the face. (a) At beginning of TCM, showing severe oozing, crust, redness, and excoriation. (b) 2 weeks of TCM. (c) 1 month of TCM, showing mild to moderate improvement. (d) 2 months of TCM, showing marked improvement.

triple TCM therapy. At the second consult, after 2 weeks of TCM, her face started to heal slightly. It improved markedly at 1 month of TCM. At 2 months, her facial lesions were nearly completely improved. Her sleep and itching also improved. Her overall SCORAD reduced to 17.2 (over 80% improved). Her lesions on other part of the body, including neck, back of the knee, behind the ear, and inner elbow were also improved by 80–90% (not shown).

In summary, this case represents rapid improvement in a young child whose symptoms were like Type I eczema. Although the skin lesions looked very severe, they responded to the TCM regimen quickly. The plan is that she will continue on phase I protocol for an additional 3 months. The key is to prevent flares. If her skin continues to improve in the following 3 months, she will complete her first milestone and transition to phase II protocol.

Type IV. Newborn Eczema and Senior Eczema

Eczema has strong genetic association. In general, the newborns will be at risk if their parents or siblings have/had eczema. I had the opportunity to see newborns with eczema (within 6 months) because I had treated their older siblings. In these families, when newborns start to show eczema, the parents seek care with me in addition to their other standard care. The treatment with newborns is only external and most of time it is sufficient. In general, their eczema will be improved within 2–4 weeks. Since the TCM regimen has shown a high safety profile, as discussed in our previous publications,[4,5] and has been used historically for newborn eczema in TCM practice in China and other Asian countries, early introduction may preclude the need for strong medication and possibly prevent the continuation of the allergy march.

In addition, there are also senior patients with recalcitrant eczema who received TCM therapy. Some of these individuals had been on chronic topical/oral steroids prior to TCM. The TCM treatment strategy would be different from other types of eczema, and patients responded well to the protocol and could achieve the healing milestones. A successful case is presented in the interviews to follow.

Overall Treatment Protocol

The triple TCM therapy protocol, including internal teas (Shi Zhen Teas), external herbal bath (Herbal Bath Additive formulations) and external creams (Herbal Cream Ia/IO) has been described in detail in our publications[4,5] and in Chapter 3 of this book. Additional experience indicates that in more severe cases, such as steroid withdrawal syndrome, freshly prepared herbal teas and customized formulation may be used.

The mechanisms of actions underlying the clinical effects may be associated with reduction or normalization of peripheral blood eosinophils and total IgE levels. Laboratory study showed that the internal tea (Shi Zhen Tea, SZT) has inhibitory effect on IL-4 production by a Th2 cell line, suppression of IgE production by human B cell line, TNF-a production by murine macrophage cell line, and exotaxin product by fibroblasts.[2-5,8] Using network pharmacology and computational modeling, we have revealed interesting molecular targets that are specific to the SZT efficacy.[2] For example, in addition to suppressing inflammatory genes, the compounds cynarine, stigmasterin, and kushenol promote anti-inflammatory genes such as peroxisome proliferator activated receptor c (PPAR c) and vitamin D receptor (VDR) that play important roles in wound healing and skin integrity. Research is underway to further understand the mechanisms and establish quantitative biomarkers to evaluate skin integrity.

All individual herbs in the triple therapy have long human-use history. Product quality control has been well established using high-performance liquid chromatography (HPLC). Based on the animal study, SZT showed high safety profile. No abnormalities were observed after feeding 10X effective dose (see Chapter 7 of this book). Clinical observation data also showed high safety data.[4] In my practice, I have also developed protocols to help individuals slowly introduce the triple therapy, particularly for very sensitive individuals, and continue to monitor their safety. Further studies on safety and efficacy are on the way.

Expected Milestones of Healing Process

There are 4 phases of treatment strategies and healing milestones (Fig. 12.7).

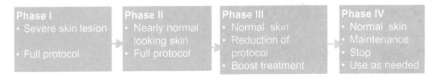

Figure 12.7.   Treatment phases. This represents the healing milestones.

- **Phase I.** Skin lesions are very severe. Individuals need full triple therapy protocol, i.e., two type of internal teas, herbal bath additive, and two different types of creams. In general, the expected milestones are: at first month, only slight sign of improvement; in 3 months, you may see moderate improvement; by 6 months of treatment, the skin lesions should be mostly improved. However, some individuals could achieve the milestone in less than 6 months, while others require more time. In this phase the difficult timeline is the first 3 months because the improvement is not stable yet. Some days may be very good, but others not. The key is to keep the protocol consistent.

- **Phase II.** Once the skin lesion stabilizes and continues to improve, the phase I milestone will be completed and transition to phase II commences. In this phase, the skin care regimen may be the same, but for a different purpose. It is to further improve the skin integrity and build a healthy skin barrier and strong platform to prepare for phase III — reduction of the regime. This phase will also start to help other co-morbid conditions. The goal in this phase is to achieve at least 3 months without any flares. This phase looks easy, but the major challenge is adherence to an admittedly demanding regime. Once skin looks and feels good, human nature is to take it easy. In addition, most herbal creams have different colors, connoting a particular sequence of use, but some age groups tend not to use them in the directed order. Additionally, severe eczema affects the vigor of children's play, but once they are better, they like to play hard. However, restraint is advisable because many of them also have systemic inflammation. Exposure to harsh environments and excessive exertion may trigger environmental allergy or asthma. This caution should also apply to adults and older children.

- **Phase III.** Once the skin is very stable without any issue for 3–6 months, or longer, the phase III protocol will start. This is the reduction protocol, including lowering cream and pill loads and starting to reduce frequency of medication days, gradually tapering to few days on the regimen while skin remains stable.

- **Phase IV.** This is to prepare to completely stop the herbal regimen. There will be no routine treatment. However, use-as-needed protocol should be available in case some harsh environment triggers skin irritation. In that instance, 1–2 weeks of intensive treatment is needed to ease the irritation.

Clinical Research

The goal is to conduct clinical research to support the safety and efficacy of TCM in patients with severe eczema and to study the mechanisms underlying its efficacy.

The FDA has allowed real-world evidence studies since 2018. We have pursued a practice-based clinical study entitled "Biomarker study of TCM effect on skin microbiota and integrity in association with the clinical scores in eczema". In this study, we will use non-invasive approach to measure skin integrity by measuring transepidermal water loss (TEWL). We will also determine skin bacterial community and gut bacteria profile, and determine their association with skin improvement, evaluated by SCORAD. Together it will allow us to quantitatively measure skin barrier/integrity.

We will conduct two cohorts:

- Cohort #1: 6 months to 4 year olds, steroid dependent, used steroid within 3 months (Type I eczema).
- Cohort #2: Adults with steroid withdrawal syndrome, Type II eczema (will also add children with ages >1 year)

Each cohort will include 40 study subjects. We have received New York Medical College Institutional Review Board (IRB) approval and are in the process of beginning the study.

Acknowledgements

Many thanks to the team and collaborators: Kamal Srivastava, PhD, Nan Yang, PhD, Raj Tiwari PhD, Jan Geliebter PhD at New York Medical College; Anna Nowak-Wegrzyn, MD, PhD at New York University; Erin Thanik, MD, Danna Chung, MD, Anne Maitland, MD, PhD, Hugh Sampson, MD at Icahn School of Medicine at Mount Sinai; Julia Wisniewski, MD at University Of Virginia Medical Center, Qian Yuan, MD, PhD at MassGeneral Hospital for Children, and Paul M. Ehrlich, MD at New York University. Thanks also to Augustine Moscatello, MD, PhD Chairman of Otolaryngology at New York Medical College for his support of integrative medicine, practice and research. Big thanks to Mrs. Kyrie Stillman for her early support and inspiration. Many special thanks to the families and patients for their hard work and support.

Disclosure

Xiu-Min Li received research support from the National Institutes of Health (NIH)/National Center for Complementary and Alternative Medicine (NCCAM); Food Allergy Research and Education (FARE) and Winston Wolkoff Integrative Medicine Fund for Allergies and Wellness; received consultancy fees from FARE and Johnson & Johnson Pharmaceutical Research & Development, L.L.C. Bayer HealthCare LLC; Received grant from Henan University of Chinese Medicine & New York Medica College for TCM Immunopharmacology and Integrative Medicine; received royalties from UpToDate; received travel expenses from the NCCAM and FARE; is an honorary professor of Henan University of Chinese Medicine, Henan, China and an honorary professor of China Medical University, Taichung, Taiwan; received practice compensation from the Integrative Health and Acupuncture PC, and US Times Technology Inc is managed by a related party; is a member of Herbs Springs, LLC, Health Freedom LLC, and General Nutraceutical Technology LLC.

References

1. Montes-Torres A, Llamas-Velasco M, Pérez-Plaza A, Solano-López G, Sánchez-Pérez J. Biological treatments in atopic dermatitis. *J Clin Med.* Apr 2015;4(4):593–613. doi:10.3390/jcm4040593
2. Wang ZZ, Jia Y, Srivastava KD, Huang W, Raj Tiwari, Nowak-Wegrzyn A, Geliebter J, Miao M and Li X-M. Systems pharmacology and in silico docking analysis to uncover association of CA2, PPARG, RXRA, and VDR with the mechanisms underlying the Shi Zhen Tea formula effect on eczema. *Evid Based Complement Alternat Med.* 2021;2021:8406127. doi:10.1155/2021/8406127
3. Srivastava K, Yang N, Uzun S, Thanik E, Ehrlich P, Chung D, Yuan Q, Nowak-Wegrzyn A, Li X-M. Effect of Traditional Chinese Medicine (TCM) in moderate-to-severe eczema in clinic and animal model: beyond corticosteroids. *J Allergy Clin Immunol.* 2020;145:AB198.

4. Wang Z, Wang ZZ, Geliebter J, Tiwari R, Li XM. Traditional Chinese medicine for food allergy and eczema. *Ann Allergy Asthma Immunol.* Dec 10 2020;doi:10.1016/j.anai. 2020.12.002

5. Thanik E, Wisniewski JA, Nowak-Wegrzyn A, Sampson H, Li XM. Effect of traditional Chinese medicine on skin lesions and quality of life in patients with moderate to severe eczema. *Ann Allergy Asthma Immunol.* Jul 2018;121(1):135–136. doi:10.1016/j.anai.2018.03.004

6. Holland SM, DeLeo FR, Elloumi HZ, *et al.* STAT3 mutations in the hyper-IgE syndrome. *N Engl J Med.* 2007/10/18 2007;357(16):1608–1619. doi:10.1056/NEJMoa073687

7. Mogensen TH. STAT3 and the hyper-IgE syndrome: Clinical presentation, genetic origin, pathogenesis, novel findings and remaining uncertainties. *JAKSTAT.* 1 Apr 2013;2(2):e23435.

8. Wisniewski J OM, Nowak-Wegrzyn A, Steenburgh-Thanik E, Sampson H, Li XM. Efficacy and safety of traditional Chinese medicine for treatment of atopic dermatitis (AD). *J Allergy Clin Immunol (Abstract).* 2010;123(2):S37.

"SHE LEARNED TO CHEW THROUGH HER SLEEVES TO GET AT HER SKIN"

Jane

Alicia (Jane's mother)

Jane began to show signs of eczema at two months, mostly in the form of very dry skin starting on her face. A succession of moisturizers only seemed to make it worse. "We tried every cream under the sun," Alicia says. Hydrocortisone helped temporarily, although Alicia read about steroids and was wary of overuse.

When Jane was six or seven months, the family visited Italy where Jane reacted badly to eating some baby food that contained wheat. A local allergist tested her and verified wheat allergy. She recommended cortisone pills, which disappointed Alicia. Alicia says that there was a family history of psoriasis in Italy, where her aunt scratched badly enough that her bloody sheets had to be changed.

Following their return to California, Jane was diagnosed with allergy to egg, sesame, soy, and oatmeal as well as wheat, and they began a course of sublingual immunotherapy for some of them.

The eczema came back. Jane was scratching all day long and had to be watched to restrain her. "We couldn't leave her alone. She learned to chew through her sleeves to get at her skin. She never oozed. It was a dry, red itch." One small blessing was that Jane slept normally. More blood tests were done, revealing sensitivity to additional foods. She didn't like solid foods and on one doctor's recommendation they rotated her on different milks, such as goat and soy, and formulas including Neocate, which is hydrolyzed. After three months, they returned to cow's milk, which was the most agreeable.

At the age of 11 months, they found Dr. Xiu-Min Li. It took about four weeks to find the right protocol. After four months of treatment, Jane's IgE levels had fallen by 50%. Her itching had stopped, and her skin's appearance was normal.

14

ECZEMATOUS LESIONS SPREAD "LIKE IVY"

Moira (Age 45)

Moira was born in Scotland and led a peripatetic life both before and after marriage. At age five, she started having atopic diseases such as asthma and environmental allergies, including to her grandparents' dog. Eczema began at eight with patches behind her knees and in the creases of her elbows. The combination of disorders would keep her out of school for a week at a time. She had terribly chapped lips.

In the UK, the National Health Service is built around general practitioners, with very few allergists available. She had allergic shiners — dark circles under the eyes that are byproducts of environmental allergies — but no one picked up on it. The only treatment for her eczema was hydrocortisone and emollients. By the time Moira reached her late teens, the eczema began to appear in patches on her face and her body. A dermatologist introduced her to light therapy, which provided some relief. After reaching university, she came to rely on daily hydrocortisone, but it did nothing to halt the spread of her eczema. With the stress of her teacher training, the eczematous lesions spread "like ivy".

She was patch tested for chemical sensitivity and bandages impregnated with corticosteroids were applied every few days at a hospital. She continued to receive light therapy.

After university, she and her husband, who was involved in international media, went on a long adventure that took them to Latin America and South Asia. She managed her skin with a combination of anti-malarial drugs and the antibiotic doxycycline, although the caution that she should avoid direct sunlight presented a problem. Upon arriving in New Zealand, she stopped taking the drugs and began to experience the "worst flares" as well as chronic sleeplessness.

They moved to Sydney where once again she was treated with hydrocortisone and more light therapy. Two years later they relocated to London. She was 35 and pregnant.

During delivery, her hands, which had never suffered before, started itching terribly. Over time it got much worse. When she resumed teaching, she went to school with her hands bandaged, and her students would ask her what was wrong. Topical steroids failed to help, and a new dermatologist recommended oral steroids. In the meantime, her son was diagnosed with food allergies. They went to one of the eminent food allergy researchers in London who gave her the name of Dr. Xiu-Min Li.

Once again, her husband's work took them abroad, this time to China. Her son's food allergies became worse, and the eczema, which had been "livable", took a bad turn with the appearance of a new trigger — perspiring. This led to her first experience with herbal medicine, although administered by a Western practitioner. MDs in China are trained in both medical traditions.

The next stop was a suburb of New York City where another pregnancy resulted in a full-body rash. A nearby "integrative" doctor performed patch testing for various antigens and started her on sublingual immunotherapy.

In 2019, her son was seeing a doctor at the Jaffe Food Allergy Institute. In July, he referred Moira to an eminent dermatologist for her eczema, which by then was on her hands, legs, and back. This doctor was conducting a clinical trial to see if an established psoriasis drug might also be effective for eczema. But not in Moira's case. Within four days she experienced flaking skin on her face, which also burned and hived. She was switched to dupilumab, the first monoclonal antibody for eczema. She found that she was gaining weight, growing sluggish, the consistency of her hair began to change and then started falling out. The hair loss was too great an indignity and she decided to quit dupilumab.

Another dermatologist near her home offered her UV light treatment, which she accepted, but wanted to put her on oral steroids, which she refused. Over a period of a few months from December 2019 to February 2020, her condition didn't seem to be getting any worse, but any improvement was very slow. Unfortunately, the COVID-19 pandemic intervened, and she stopped going. From March to July, "I was living on antihistamines." Her eyebrows fell out. She drank for the pain. Her husband was trying to work and parent the kids. Finally, she looked up a name she had heard 10 years before from her allergist in the UK — Dr. Li. On a Facebook page, she saw the case of a boy whose terrible eczema had been successfully treated (see Chapter 12 of this book). Dr. Li studied Moira's test results and asked her to stop eating a few foods and put her on her protocol. Within a week she was sleeping through the night and had stopped itching.

15

THEY SWADDLED HIM AT NIGHT AND RESTRAINED HIS HANDS WITH VELCRO

Artie (Age 2½)

Carol (Artie's mother)

Artie started to show eczema on his cheeks at three months. First a pediatrician and then a dermatologist recommended using hydrocortisone. Carol, Artie's mother, was a post-partum nurse and wary of steroids, but she followed the prescription. The eczema rapidly spread to the rest of his body and the backs of his legs started "weeping". At the age of nine months, he was diagnosed with allergies to several foods including eggs, fish, and soy.

Artie needed round-the-clock attention to comfort him and stop him from scratching. The smallest scratch would produce "a lot of blood". At every opportunity, he would scratch his face till it bled. They swaddled him at night and restrained his hands with Velcro, but he learned to flip himself over and rub his face. His bedding needed laundering every day to get the blood out. The car seat was also bloody, and they had to strap Artie's hands with more Velcro. They bathed him in sea salt, bathed him with bleach, and tried whatever other ideas they could find on the internet or from their doctors. When Artie was one, a holistic practitioner mentioned Dr. Li, but it would be a year before they consulted her.

Eventually the pressure became too much. Carol's job required that she spend her nights at the hospital. The experience of caring for other people's children overnight while her son needed her "made me feel like I was crazy". She and her husband took a dramatic leap: Carol quit her job and they sold their house.

Carol continued to comb the internet for ideas. Eventually she came across some before-and-after pictures on Facebook posted by another mother. The progress recorded after just two weeks of treatment for a child whose condition was similar to Artie's was enough to convince Carol and her husband, so they took some of the proceeds from the sale of their house and started working with Dr. Li. After a month, there were no open wounds or weeping. After two months, Artie could wear short-sleeved shirts.

16

"I WOULD OOZE AND CRY"

Ellen

The problem began when her sister recommended a "non-steroidal" house-branded face cream from a salon in Manhattan, which she used twice a day for 15 years, starting in her late 20s. During that time the product grew in fame and became a big seller on Amazon. The marketing reach spread to South Korea, which, Ellen says, tests cosmetics as well as pharmaceuticals and the cream was found to be 70% steroidal. As the Amazon reviews switched from positive to negative, Ellen began suffering symptoms of topical steroid addiction, and then withdrawal.

Ellen suffered from shakes as her adrenal system malfunctioned and her skin looked like second degree burns. She developed MRSA (Methicillin-resistant *Staphylococcus aureus*) on her face and other staph infections on her legs. The crooks of her elbows were so badly affected that she couldn't bend her arms fully or straighten them. "Oozing smells," she says.

But the worst of it was the pain. Ellen says, "I had a nine-pound baby and it was nothing like this. I would ooze and cry. I took Lyrica for nerve pain, hydroxyzine for itching and to help me sleep, valium for anxiety, oxycodone for general pain and assorted antibiotics for my infections." She credits her husband for keeping her to the prescribed frequency for the opioids because she wanted them every 20 minutes. She took long Epsom salt baths. She also kept a rotation of ice packs going with the help of her son who called himself the ice-pack jockey. Ellen says the packs only stayed cold enough to do her any good for seven minutes and then had to go back in the freezer. Her doctors were no help. One said, "These things happen." And another said she should go to the emergency room. No acknowledgement of topical steroid addiction or withdrawal. She was given oxycodone and valium.

The low point of the multi-year ordeal was a 48-hour period when she couldn't get off the couch. At midnight one night, she called her best friend and asked her if she could come over and take care of her son while her husband took her to the ER, and there was a period when her parents took over childcare altogether. She barely left home from June to October 2017, and when she did, disguised herself with big hats and sunglasses.

Finally, Ellen came across a documentary on Google about red skin and topical steroid withdrawal showing Dr. Li and the arm of a patient, before and after. She immediately recognized her condition and contacted Dr. Li's office. In her first appointment in June 2017, Dr. Li reassured her and gave her acupuncture to relieve pain and anxiety, and Ellen left with some measure of hope. The following September she felt presentable enough to take her son to his first day of kindergarten. After a year, she felt strong enough to appear at a conference to give an account of her experience to an audience of doctors and lay people. As of this writing, it has been two years and while she has occasional flares, it is nothing like before.

And she is part of a lawsuit against the company that sold the cream as steroid free.

17

"WHEN WE WERE LITTLE, YOUR SKIN SCARED ME"

Ava (Age 20)

While Ava was at summer camp in her mid-teens, she met a girl from her home town. The girl said, "When we were little, your skin scared me." Hearing this hurt, but Ava understood. She had been a patient of Dr. Li starting at age 13.

She was born with eczema. Her pediatric dermatologist tried every topical steroid, but nothing was long-term effective. She tried light therapy, which had no effect. Finally, the dermatologist suggested going to see Dr. Li, which was remarkable since Dr. Li hadn't been in practice very long and most of her patients arrived via word of mouth from colleagues in New York City — Ava lived in a suburb.

She recalls that her skin itched behind her knees and in the crooks of her elbows. Her hands were dry and bled from scratching. Her skin was so dry, it would just spontaneously split, particularly in hot weather. Her bedsheets were bloody. When she watched television in the family living room, she lay on a towel.

She understood her friend's comment about scary skin. When her class had exercises that involved holding hands and standing in a circle, she would apologize and explain. To scratch her back, Ava would find a surface to rub, like the bark of trees and doorways.

Her first visit with Dr. Li was "overwhelming". It was in New York City and she had to take a whole afternoon. Clinic was held on Saturdays, but because Ava and other patients were observant Jews, Dr. Li held clinic on Wednesdays to accommodate them. The initial treatment involved swallowing "gross tea", which she refused to swallow. Dr. Li reformulated the tea into pills.

After treatment began, her life changed. Instead of asking why her hands were dry and bloody, her classmates would ask why they were blue — stained by the creams. She rapidly improved, and while treatment is now in its 8th year, she has occasional bouts of dry skin. But the itching is gone. Ava no longer thinks about her skin all the time.

18

"EVEN THE AIR HURT HIS SKIN"

Josh (Age 12)

Susan (Josh's mother)

Josh had suffered from eczema since birth. Over seven years, he had count-less applications of steroid creams and at least 12–15 rounds of oral steroids. When he began kindergarten in August of 2014, his parents realized his skin had stopped responding to their normal protocol. Topical steroids no longer helped his flares. Only oral steroids brought any relief at all. His parents then noticed that after each course of steroids, his flares would come back worse.

By the start of 1st grade (Aug 2015), his entire world began to shift. Each night he would "shed an entire layer of skin". His bed would be cov-ered in it. Susan says, "He would walk out of his room oozing and in extreme pain. I took him to countless doctors and hospitals. The hospitals would just tell me that this was the most severe case they had seen and give us another round of steroids and ask us to follow up with allergists… His oral steroids would be followed by EXTREME flares days later." No one knew what to do. His food allergies were "snow balling". He was allergic to milk, eggs, soy, wheat, shellfish, peanuts, and tree nuts.

During Christmas of 2015, Josh had to be pulled temporarily from school because "even the air hurt his skin". He sat on the couch for hours with a quilt over his head with the IPad. He was unable to play with his brothers and rarely smiled. The family confined their activity to their house and Susan says, "Life became very dark." New tests showed sensitivity to environmental allergens, notably dog dander and dust mites. The day they got the results, they got rid of all cloth-upholstered furniture and found a new home for Josh's beloved dog. Replacing the furniture with leather was easy enough but comforting a very broken-hearted little boy who missed his dog was much more difficult.

Susan says, "I continued searching for answers and took him to several doctors. The only answer anyone could give me was steroids. We knew steroids were only temporary and meant massive flares after." She and her husband resolved to throw way all topical steroids and refused oral steroids. She says now that she knows this was NOT the way to do it but their experience had been so bad, they were feeling desperate. Things went from bad to worse. She stopped taking Josh to medical appointments and asked her husband to go in her place. "Doctors seemed to be blaming me for not following protocol. I felt they believed maybe I was mistreating him. It was just better for everyone for my husband to take him."

Once they took Josh back to Children's Healthcare of Atlanta Emergency Room. Again, the doctors only offered steroids, and recommended follow up with the family allergist. "I drove straight to his office," says Susan. "Josh still had on his hospital bracelet." She demanded to speak with the allergist right away. "I was holding a little boy who had trouble walking and his skin was falling off." The doctor pulled up a chair and asked her if she was open to different types of treatment. "EXTREMELY open." He told Susan of Dr. Li and her work. He told her that he would have a mother who had a child in treatment call her. "When I left the appointment, the mother called right away. I sat in the parking lot talking to her for about 30 minutes."

It took a few months to get an appointment. During this time Josh suffered several flares. He begged to attend school a few hours a day. He said he thought he could make it until 11:15. "He loved school and had made up his mind that this was his goal. The school was very cooperative in general. His favorite teacher, who recognized the potential for disruption Josh's condition presented, told the class that it showed how devoted he was to school and that students should be supportive. The school nurses gave him his antihistamines. He took four doses of hydroxyzine and two of ibuprofen daily. He also took ceterizine. He came home and showered immediately, then got back under his quilt." Josh, now 12, says school was a distraction from his pain.

A week before their June 1, 2016 appointment with Dr. Li in New York City, Josh started to become very ill. He developed an oozing rash. They visited a walk-in clinic and two hospitals during that week. The doctors believed he had impetigo and a staph infection. Josh was given a shot of steroids along with antibiotics to help make it through the two-day drive to New York, which they thought was necessary because Josh's appearance would alarm other passengers if they flew. Josh, now 12, remembers it as "long, boring, and painful". His dad had to clean the crust on his eyelids so he could see.

When they arrived at Dr. LI's office, Josh couldn't walk, could barely talk, and his eyelids had crusted shut again. Dr. Li examined him and asked that they also see an allergist (Dr. Paul Ehrlich) to evaluate whether or not Josh could begin treatment or if he would require hospitalization. Dr. Ehrlich carried Josh into his consulting room and also asked a dermatologist whose office was down the hall to weigh in. They applied some topical antibiotics and assured the family that they were in good hands with Dr. Li. Susan asked the allergist if he had any advice. He simply said, "Do everything she tells you." They had to boil and prepare the herbs for each bath. He required creams every 2 hours and took 90 total pills daily. "This kid was determined and did not complain. He knew it was working so that motivated him. We set timers and made it a point to give thanks to Dr Li and the treatment."

Josh began to improve rapidly, and family quality of life improved with it. Now at age 12, Josh is articulate, happy, and itch free.

Postscript

The following is adapted from a clinical write-up of this case in the form of a published letter entitled "Improvement of skin lesions in corticosteroid addiction/withdrawal-associated severe eczema by combined traditional Chinese medicine" written by Serife Uzun, MS, Zixi Wang, MD, Tory A McKnight (medical student), Paul Ehrlich, MD, Erin Thanik, MD, Anna Nowak-Wegrzyn, MD, Nan Yang, PhD, and Xiu-Min Li, MD:

Here, we present the case of a highly allergic pediatric patient with steroid-refractory chronic AD and steroid addiction/withdrawal syndrome who was successfully treated with multi-component TCM therapy.

A 6-year-old male with atopic dermatitis (AD) since 2 months of life presents with persistent refractory AD despite chronic mid-potency topical corticosteroid use and an 18-month trial of step-up therapy to high-potency topical corticosteroids. Prior to TCM, over a 6-month period, he had used 8 courses of oral prednisone treatment to control his eczema (5 days/course). However, the eczematous lesions returned as soon as 3 days after completing the last course of prednisone, and progressed to total body erythroderma over 12 days, more severe compared to that prior to prednisone use. He was diagnosed with steroid-withdrawal syndrome with the complication of *Staphylococcus aureus* infection confirmed by skin culture. He responded poorly to antibiotics (oral cephalexin and topical mupirocin) combined with steroid injection. He was referred to the senior author by his primary allergist, secondary allergist, and dermatologist for trial of TCM therapy at the Integrative Health and Acupuncture PC in New York. Upon the first visit for TCM therapy in June 2016, the patient presented with total body erythroderma characterized further by severe erythema, edema, oozing, and excoriations as well as extensive blistering and bleeding (see Fig. 12.4(a)). Disease was severe based on a score of 103 by standardized SCORAD. He was unable to walk secondary to pain and had daytime somnolence related to restless sleep. His medical history was significant for multiple food allergies and allergic rhinitis associated with perennial and seasonal allergen sensitization. Despite taking cetirizine, diphenhydramine and hydroxyzine, he reported uncontrollable pruritus. Laboratory results provided by his primary allergist indicated elevated total serum IgE (19,000 kIU/L, normal 100kIU/L), eosinophilia (1×10^3 cells/μL, normal range 0–0.3 $\times$ 10^3 cells/μL), and high specific IgE levels to multiple food and environmental allergens (see Table 12.1). His Aspartate Aminotransferase (AST), Alanine Transaminase (ALT) and Blood Urea Nitrogen (BUN) levels were all within normal range (see Table 12.1).

The patient received combined TCM therapy of Herbal Bath Additive, Herbal Creams and internal tea, described previously. Within one week of treatment, his lesions showed signs of improvement (see Fig. 12.4(b)). By 1 month of treatment, his skin lesion intensity was significantly improved;

there was no oozing, erythema, or excoriation, with persistence of dryness and lichenification (see Fig. 12.4(c)). His SCORAD values decreased by 79% (from 103 to 21.8) after 1 month of TCM and by 99% following 6 months of TCM (see Fig. 12.4(e)). Most strikingly, he showed rapid improvement in his quality of sleep within one week and the patient reported no itching by two weeks of treatment. Notably, throughout TCM treatment, he did not require use of oral or topical steroids. His total serum IgE decreased 75% (from 19,000 kIU/L to 4,630 kIU/L) by 12 months (see Table 12.1). Absolute eosinophil counts decreased by 60% (from 1×10^3 to 0.427×10^3 cells/μL). Liver and kidney function tests remained within normal range (see Table 12.1). His skin remained well controlled while on maintenance of TCM regimen, and by 17 months of TCM, he was able to taper and discontinue the TCM regimen without any flare-up. His skin continued to be well controlled 3 months after discontinuation of TCM (see Fig. 12.4(f)).

In summary, we present a case of steroid-withdrawal syndrome treated with combined TCM in a 6-year-old child with chronic AD since infancy. Several of the herbs used in this case study have known immunologic effects. The active component of *Radix arnebiae* is Shikonin, which has been shown to reduce TGF-β-induced collagen production in scar-derived fibroblasts. *Radix glycyrrhizae* has been shown to inhibit LPS induced NF-κB activation, a key player in AD disease pathology, and its compound 7,4 dihydroxyflavone reduces eotaxin-production and Th2 cytokines. *Kochia scopariae*-derived oleanolic acid demonstrated antibiotic properties against *Listeria monocytogenes*. *Flos lonicerae* has antibacterial action against *Staphlococcus aureus*, streptococci, and *Salmonella typhi*, and exhibits an anti-inflammatory effect and hepatic cell protective effect. In this case study, the mechanisms of action were not studied, however, the combined herbal approach allows for utilization of the anti-inflammatory and anti-microbial properties of these key herbs. In vitro studies have shown that the herbal internal tea used for this patient has anti-IgE, eotaxin, and TNF-α effects (data not shown). Previous study showed it inhibited Th2 cytokine IL-4 production. More studies are needed to investigate the combined effects of the components of the integrated TCM for AD. Large studies are needed to confirm the efficacy of this combined TCM for steroid-withdrawal in patients with chronic AD and steroid addiction.

Photographs of Josh on the Day He Began Treatment

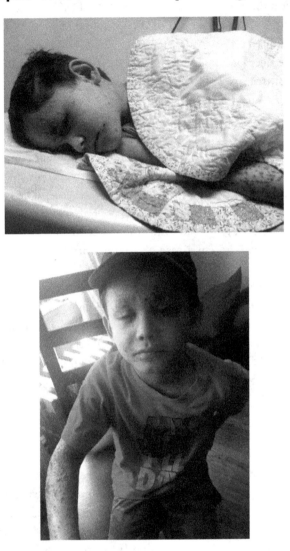

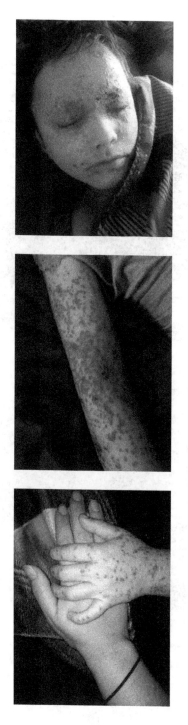

Photographs of Josh After 3 Months of Treatment

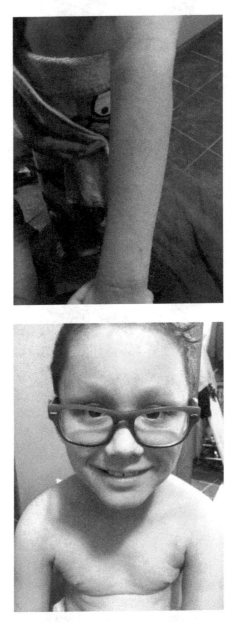

Photographs of Josh at End of Treatment After 18 Months

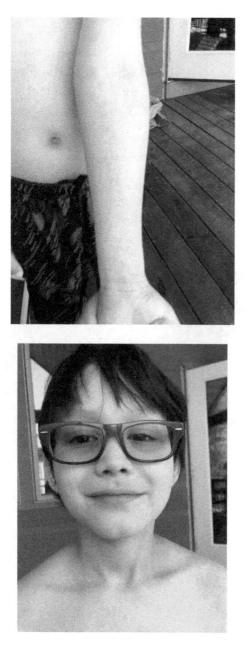

THE CONDITION LOOKED LIKE ECZEMA BUT IT "BEHAVED DIFFERENTLY"

Gladys (Age 83)

Gladys is Josh's grandmother. She also lives in Georgia, near enough to Josh and his family to have been very supportive in his treatment.

Gladys was born in Alaska. She is a full-blooded member of the Tlingit tribe. She grew up in a village where Indians, Eskimos, Filipinos, and whites lived poor-but-happy lives. They ate fresh fish and seal cooked with seal oil, ate locally grown vegetables, and spent many hours picking wild berries. Like many native Americans, she was not so happy with being sent away to boarding schools where she lost touch with her tribal language and customs.

She remembers being very itchy from an early age, a problem her government-sponsored health care couldn't resolve. She was given salves. After high school, she studied to be a dental hygienist. She worked first in an Indian hospital and later at a private practice in Seattle where she met and married Harold, Susan's father, who was in the Navy. After he left the service, they moved to Georgia. During all of this, she continued to suffer from skin problems. A dermatologist told her the condition looked like eczema but it "behaved differently". She used a succession of steroidal and nonsteroidal creams. In the last few years, an allergist suggested dupilumab, which had just come to market.

Eventually, Susan brought up the possibility of Dr. Li's treatment. Gladys and Harold were well acquainted with it because of Josh's experience. They had assisted in his treatment. The doctors were agreeable. Harold was also agreeable because he had been treated for a gastric ailment with Chinese herbal tea in Hong Kong during his military service.

Dr. Li had never had a patient of Gladys's age. Younger patients have malleable immune systems. She gave Gladys a very thorough examination and various salves and pills. She made a slow steady progress while being tapered off her other medications, with regular phone consultations with Dr. Li, initially every two weeks and later every month.

Gladys's Hands Before and After Treatment

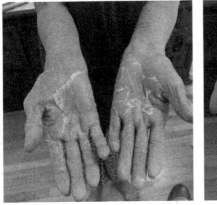 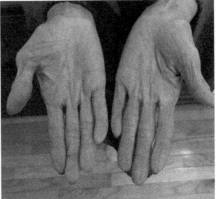

20

A "BLUR OF MISERY"

Lawrence (Age 7½)

Molly (Lawrence's mother)

Lawrence's eczema started at four months. A dermatologist recommended low-steroid creams and ointments but said it would be a year before he would be able to make any judgment about the condition possibly resolving on its own. It didn't and the dermatologist recommended a stronger steroid, which did help.

Lawrence had some hives, and the pediatrician recommended testing for food allergies, which showed sensitivity to dairy and eggs. Molly was still breastfeeding and removed these foods from her diet, which did help, although after a few days away from home, during which she ate both, the hives returned.

The eczema worsened. The parents installed a baby monitor and watched him scratch until he fell asleep. They tried special pajamas, but they didn't work. "Wet wraps only made him cry," says Molly. Looking back, she described this period as a "blur of misery". Touching Lawrence's skin made her feel deeply sad. "It was like fragile paper… When I saw him touch it, I would jump to attention. He was always scratching and I would say 'please stop.'"

At age three, an allergist tried some low-steroid creams again, which seemed to help. They also discussed food allergies. By then Lawrence had suffered two episodes of anaphylaxis from milk exposure. His lips began to swell and Molly promptly administered epinephrine. Along the way, symptoms of asthma began to appear, often triggered by colds. Albuterol was given as needed, although there was one scare when Lawrence contracted enterovirus, which was going around. He spent three days in the hospital. At age five, the allergist brought up Dr. Li's name, but Molly said that she forgot about it for a few months until the pediatrician, who practiced at Mt. Sinai, also suggested Dr. Li. They made an appointment for June 2017.

Dr. Li's first reaction was how fragile Lawrence looked. Molly says, "This was an eye opener because when you see your child every day, you get used to his appearance." They created a plan to treat the eczema first because it causes day-to-day suffering, and when it was controlled, to go after the food allergies. Dr. Li seemed confident that he would make rapid progress. She gave him acupressure, which seemed to help. Lawrence slept better that night. He took the baths and the creams well. The oral teas were a bit of a challenge because he had never swallowed a capsule, and they were too bitter to dissolve in juice, but hiding them in applesauce worked. His eczema was undetectable in a few months. Oddly, he began to get a few hives now and then, which mystified Mom, but Dr. Li said that this was a good sign because previously Lawrence's skin was too frail to form hives. Lawrence himself figured out the source. He said they only came up when he was getting ready to go out, or otherwise getting excited.

At this telling, after two years of treatment, Lawrence's total IgE has fallen from 3900 to 439. He has used no albuterol for a year, growth is normal, general health is far better — no more coughs and colds — and "his skin is great".

"THIS WAS NO WAY TO LIVE"

Alex (Age 11)

Janet (Alex's mother)

Alex began to show signs of eczema at the age of three weeks and the pediatrician recommended topical steroids. Because his two older siblings had food allergies, the parents consulted an allergist, although he declined to test for specific allergies right away. Alex's condition deteriorated substantially. He and his mother Janet were down to only two hours of sleep a night. She nursed him for hours at a time and held his hands to keep him from scratching, sometimes futilely. Once she woke up and her shirt was soaked with pus from an infected cheek.

Janet was trained as a bio-chemist and her husband is a polymer chemist. They were accustomed to seeking and finding solutions to problems, which made their experience with MDs more frustrating. Alex had seven anaphylactic reactions in all. He also had asthma severe enough to require hospitalization. Told by an allergist to avoid 45 foods, she decided, "This was no way to live. He was crying. I was crying. I stopped nursing." Her son was subsisting on white rice and sweet potatoes. He was dehydrated. His skin was weepy and infected. He was taking hydroxyzine, antibiotics, and oral steroids. She started doing her own research.

One night she was prowling the internet and came across the name of Gina Clowes, who writes for *Allergic Living* and contacted her. Ms. Clowes listened to Janet's story and recommended Dr. Xiu-Min Li. She emailed Janet at 6AM with contact information, but by that time Janet already had it and had reached out to Dr. Li's research office and received a call from her assistant later in the day.

Initially, Alex and his mother flew to New York one Saturday a month for appointments. Janet says that within a few days, their sleep had improved from two hours a night to five. Within a month, the weeping and infected skin had largely resolved, although Dr. Li weaned Alex gradually off his strong medications over a year. By the age of 18 months, Alex occasionally had a spot of eczema, which could be treated with a bit of topical steroid. Today at the age of 11, he has been asthma free for five years and is down to five food allergies — chicken, sunflower seeds, and a few tree nuts.

22

POTENTIAL FOR MUCH WORSE

Geoffrey

Terry (Geoffrey's mother)

Geoffrey is the third child. The older ones have a bit of eczema but no food allergies. Terry is a physician in family practice and her husband is an emergency room doctor. At the age of a month or two, Geoffrey began to develop eczema. Terry was breastfeeding. After consulting an allergist, she stopped eating dairy, soy, and later eggs. There were many sleepless nights. They kept him covered to keep him from scratching and cut his nails every day as precautions. "We knew he wasn't severe, but knew there was potential for much worse," says Terry.

At one year, Geoffrey had a reaction to hummus and tested positive for sesame. After trying peanut butter, he had hives and swollen lips. They cut out all nuts. He reacted with hives to tomato and banana. By 18 months, they were taking out still more foods and using steroids. They were also seeing an allergist at La Crosse Associates in Wisconsin, pioneers in sublingual immunotherapy. They looked into an oral immunotherapy study at Mount Sinai but it would have required coming to New York every two or three weeks. Then Terry came across Dr. Li's name on a medical website. They had their initial appointment when Geoffrey was a bit past age two.

The initial protocol consisted of baths and creams because he had trouble with pills, but Dad taught Geoffrey to swallow them at age 2½. There was some skin improvement in the first month or two but after 6 months it was dramatically better. Terry says, "We didn't realize how bad it had been until we started with Dr. Li. We didn't really sleep before that."

In the years since, many foods have been restored to Geoffrey's diet. He also had some environmental allergies that had been treated with sublingual immunotherapy. They are notably improved.

23

ITCH THAT NEVER SEEMED TO BUDGE

Olivia Age 7

Tina (Olivia's mother)

Olivia was born with cradle cap. She was breastfed and itched extensively following feeding. In her baby photographs, she appears with socks on both hands to prevent scratching. She had extreme diaper rash. Soy and cow's milk infant formulas made her vomit, and there was an episode of anaphylaxis to dairy at three months. By six months, eczema appeared, and an infected cold sore put her in the hospital for a week.

After that, her skin would get re-infected every three weeks. Olivia was treated successively with acyclovir, a baby-dose antiviral, and triamcinolone, a topical steroid. By 18 months, she was "incredibly itchy". She would "cry and moan" and suffered from staph infections. At age two, they tried the well-known eczema treatment of Dr. Richard Aron, which combines topical steroids and antibiotics. It helped at first, but the duration of efficacy got shorter and shorter. She also developed severe asthma. Three courses of oral steroids caused Olivia's face to double in size and she stopped growing. An endocrinologist told them that this could be from the steroids, "or Olivia could just be short". The eczema spread to her scalp and she developed an antibiotic-resistant staph infection on her feet, which turned bloody. They also did photo therapy.

They decided to suspend the steroids, which suppress the immune system, and concentrate on fighting the infection, but they encountered a new symptom. Olivia's skin "turned red like sunburn". She was so sensitive she couldn't bathe. After a time, the redness went away, but she started getting chills and her skin started peeling from water loss. In September 2019 at age 4½, a dermatologist put her on cyclosporine, an immune suppressant commonly used to treat organ rejection after organ transplantation. It helped with the itching. In December Olivia was given another immune suppressant, methotrexate, also used to treat cancer and rheumatoid arthritis. Videos taken after 10 months of topical steroid withdrawal show Olivia scratching compulsively. Her mother says, "The first few months of withdrawal were brutal: oozing, chills, open skin, no sleep, and a deep and relentless itch that never seemed to budge."

They started treatment with Dr. Li in mid-September of 2020. By early December, Olivia had had no asthma for two months. After so many years of nighttime distress, she is sleeping well and when she does wake up, she isn't itching and crying. By the following March, the videos show Olivia dancing. Her mother said "Now she's feeling better than she ever did. Feeling like a little kid. It has been hard work. I hate to use the word 'miracle' but it does feel that way."

24

SHE FELT COMPLETELY HEALED, AND CELEBRATED BY GOING OUT AND DANCING UNTIL 3AM

Penny (Age 30)

Penny's problems began at two weeks of age when she broke out in hives. She had food allergies, first to dairy and grains, then found out she was allergic to eggs, when they splashed on her skin, not even ingested, and anaphylaxis to gluten. She was breastfed longer than the average child, which resulted in Lyme Disease symptoms at the age of four when her mother contracted Lyme during a trip to New York from their home in Colorado, although the disease was not yet well known (she didn't receive a definitive diagnosis until age 20). At age 5, she showed signs of depression and anxiety. Her symptoms escalated until high school when they stabilized a bit before resuming their upward trajectory.

Her skin grew sicker. Penny's mother, a nurse, steered her away from treatment with topical steroids. During high school, she was given rounds of prednisone which provided welcome relief but after a time stopped working. For five years from ages 22–27, she used steroids intensively but during the pauses she noticed signs of what she now recognizes as topical steroid withdrawal (TSW). Her eczema was aggravated by the dry air of Colorado, especially during winter.

She couldn't eat and her weight fell to 88 pounds (5'3" tall). She scratched continually to relieve the itching. In the intervals between scratching, she felt pain in her joints and muscles and what she calls zappers — cascading bursts of nerve pain at various spots on her skin. She rarely slept through the night. She lost friends as they could no longer abide her company. A bright spot — it did help her end an abusive relationship.

The misery escalated. During TSW Penny couldn't tolerate moisture. She went for long periods without bathing, although her parents helped her wash her hair. Unable to drag herself to bed, she stayed on the couch. She had trouble lifting a fork to eat, and had trouble tolerating food when her mother fed her. Her mother used silver gel to help combat patches of infection and covered the wounds with bandages infused with Manuka honey, which reportedly has antibiotic properties. She thought about suicide.

The turning point was when Nurse Mom came across two books about Dr. Xiu-Min Li. She was given an appointment promptly. She was fortified with a combination of sedating antihistamine hydroxyzine and "low-dose pig-cultured" cortisol, an anti-inflammatory, and the mast cell inhibitor sodium cromolyn, for her flight to New York. She managed to walk to the gate for her eastbound flight, although she used a wheelchair for the return.

As she embarked on treatment, Penny's thoughts were conflicted. She was optimistic but skeptical about non-Western medicine. She hadn't taken a bath for a year and a half, so she began with foot baths. Because of an allergy to corn, used in formulating herbal teas, she used a special decoction of the raw herbs as a liquid tea and sipped it over a period of hours. By six-to-eight months, she felt completely healed and celebrated by going out and dancing until 3AM.

25

"IT LOOKED LIKE SHE HAD BEEN SKINNED ALIVE FROM HEAD TO TOE"

Wendy (Age 2½)

Jeanine (Wendy's mother)

Wendy's eczema began on her cheeks when she was an infant. By age six months, it was sufficiently troubling to warrant a trip to a pediatric dermatologist who prescribed the topical steroid Mometasone, which worked initially but between applications symptoms began to escalate. White bumps appeared and by the age of one, her skin became notably lighter.

After reading about topical steroid withdrawal, Jeanine attempted to taper off Mometasone, but Wendy's skin became significantly worse. Jeanine says, "It looked like she had been skinned alive from head to toe."

The dermatologist said the escalating symptoms were from staph infection. Staph sits on the skin and when the already-delicate, itchy skin is continually scratched, the staph takes hold. Wendy was prescribed topical antibiotics on top of the steroid three times a week.

The raw oozing skin was painful. Jeanine said the only skin that was spared was the tip of Wendy's nose. The baby was still primarily breastfed, and Jeanine analyzed her own diet minutely. She experimented with supplements. Nothing helped. Family life suffered as mother and father took turns holding their child to keep her from scratching. The only way they could keep her distracted was letting her watch cartoons.

After prowling online, she came across the International Topical Steroid Addiction Network (ITSAN) and then Dr. Xiu-Min Li's practice. Since skin disorders are a priority for Dr. Li, Jeanine managed to secure an appointment for her daughter the following week, in August 2018.

Dr. Li asked her associate, a licensed allergist, to order blood tests, which revealed elevated eosinophils — high 8000 level — and IgE to a wide range of environmental and foods.

They began a regimen of raw herbs extracted by boiling into liquid because the processed teas contain corn, to which Wendy was allergic; baths twice a day and alternating 1-A and I-0 creams every two hours. By the next day, Jeanine says, there seemed to be reduced infection on the skin. By November, the skin was "half healed". By the time of this writing — April 2019 — she says Wendy is 90 percent clear, a "completely different child". She is now more interested in books than in television.

The process hasn't been easy. Jeanine has taken a leave of absence from work to ensure that her daughter's protocol could be observed on schedule, and her husband has been working overtime to pay for it, but they "got our daughter back". She is "thriving and happy".

26

SHE KEPT A DUSTBUSTER BY HER BED TO COLLECT DEAD SKIN

Nanette

Nanette's eczema began in infancy. Medical records and her mother's recollection showed it was mild until 4 to 6 months, and was accompanied by gastrointestinal problems. She was diagnosed at age two for being allergic to milk, later outgrown, and reactive to red food colorings.

Her eczema was especially bad during the winter, and steroids were applied to folds in her neck, the backs of her knees, and the creases of her elbows. At night, she wore cotton gloves and socks to minimize scratching. She avoided swimming pools and the ocean because both provoke terrible itching. She was given steroids such as halobetasol.

In 2014, Nanette experienced a terrible outbreak. New allergy tests showed sensitivity to nuts, sunflower, and peas, and patch tests showed contact dermatitis to nickel. She was admitted to a clinical trial for Apremilast, which had been certified for psoriasis and psoriatic arthritis but was being tested for other immune-mediated inflammatory disorders. She tried light therapy and another psoriasis drug called Stelara. The biologic Dupixent (dupilumab) offered some help but it also caused her hair to fall out. Nanette says, "It didn't help enough to compensate for that." She tried acupuncture. "It was relaxing but it didn't help with the underlying condition." She was very red behind her knees, elbows, and around her eyes. Her skin flaked so badly that she kept a Dustbuster by her bed to collect dead skin. Her skin was so vulnerable that when she and relatives took turns sitting vigil in the hospital room of a sick friend, Nanette was the only one who contracted scabies.

She heard about Dr. Xiu-Min Li, but after she heard a patient of Dr. Li speak at the 2018 East-West Conference at New York Medical College and spoke to the mother of another patient, she was persuaded to make an appointment, which took place on August 25. She recalled that as she got up to leave after that first appointment, Dr. Li pointed out that her pants were sticking to the backs of her legs.

With Nanette depressed and demoralized, her husband took over primary responsibility looking after their eight-year-old son. "I felt like a prisoner in my own home. It hurt to walk." She wouldn't go out.

She visited Dr. Li's clinic three weekends a month to monitor her protocol and for acupuncture. With a strict protocol of baths and two-hour applications of her creams, she received a three-month leave from her social-worker duties in a public school. As she continued to taper off her steroids, her knees would wobble.

As the treatment went on, her symptoms began to ease up and her mood lifted. She returned to her job and the students welcomed her, saying how much they missed her. That helped. Her anxiety and quality-of-life scores rose substantially. She cut down her office visits to monthly and experienced very few flares of her disease. And her medications were reduced. "I couldn't afford to keep buying new clothes." Today her skin is much better, her moods are elevated, and family life is normal.

27

"MY BABY IS GOING TO DIE IF I CAN'T HELP HIM"

Malcolm (Age 3)

Andrea (Malcolm's mother)

A few weeks after Malcolm was born, his skin turned bumpy and red. He was diagnosed with baby acne and sebaceous dermatitis before the doctor settled on eczema. Blood tests showed sensitivity to numerous foods, notably wheat and dairy, and they were removed from his diet. At age five months, an allergist was consulted, who turned out to have no experience with a child that young. A dermatologist whose manner Andrea described as condescending questioned the association with allergies, but because Malcolm's skin was "falling off" they embarked on an escalating program of topical steroids, some of which were adult strength. Malcolm was in such pain that he was delayed in sitting up.

When Malcolm was 14 months, he was getting topical steroids, "2½% on the hotspots and 1% everywhere else." He was sensitive to many foods. Exposure to perfume caused him to break out in hives. With three older brothers, managing him was very difficult, although they were protective and considerate. Andrea described his existence as "bubble-boy". There was no "happy naked-baby phase". He had to wear 100% cotton. Once when he wore a blended fabric, "he ripped it off". Scented candles and dogs caused him to tear at his skin. He was fully covered year-round and had to wear two pairs of socks at a time to contain the bleeding.

Andrea searched the internet at night looking for a doctor who could help her son. "I thought, 'my baby is going to die if I can't help him.'"

She finally found Dr. Li's name and met an allergist who had heard of her. They came from the Midwest to Dr. Li's office. Within three weeks, Malcolm's skin was "amazingly better. After three years, it is perfect. They have added numerous foods to his diet. They have lost their fear of visiting other homes. Malcolm plays with his cousins. It has been a struggle financially — Andrea has been bartending and is studying for a real estate license — but it has been worth it.

28

HE HAS BEGUN TO HAVE A NORMAL CHILDHOOD

Thomas (Age 3)

Nina (Thomas's mother)

Thomas began showing eczema symptoms at three months. The symptoms continually worsened for two and a half years. The family lives near a distinguished teaching hospital that operates a pediatric dermatology clinic. In all Thomas was seen by six dermatologists. The typical visit involved an hour or more of waiting during which Thomas would resort to scratching and was generally miserable.

The only treatment given was topical steroids in escalating strengths. While the family tried to stick to directions for on and off use, the flares were so severe during the off days that they would resort to using it on those days, too.

At night Nina slept sitting up so she could hold her son. Or she would stay awake while he slept to monitor his lesions. Thomas's skin was head-to-toe oozing, crusting, and having infections. His days were spent lying on his stomach on the couch with his iPad even after he learned to walk. He didn't play with toys. His skin oozed, sweated, and crusted. The ooze had a strongly metallic smell.

When he became infected, they would go to the doctor for antibiotics, but sometimes not fill the inevitable steroid prescriptions. He was on antibiotics for six months straight. Eventually the doctors began lobbying for oral steroids.

Finally, they started to avoid the doctors because they were exhausted from getting the same answer every time: more steroids, with the tiresome, frustrating on-again off-again directions. They stopped using steroids and Thomas exhibited signs of drug withdrawal including trembling. They returned to the clinic where a new resident appeared to be more sympathetic and proposed using Dupixent to stave off infections, off-label since it hadn't yet been approved for children that age.

Eventually Nina's research led her to Dr. Li's clinic. Within two weeks, Thomas's skin began to improve markedly. His sleep improved and he began to have a normal childhood.

29

THE MESSAGE WAS ALWAYS THE SAME. "THIS IS LIFE FOR HIM"

Charles (Age 9)

Julie (Charles's mother)

Julie says, "I felt like Charles's whole environment made him itch." She knew he needed help and felt that it "couldn't be possible for him to live in this condition forever".

She had minor eczema as a child, mostly dried, cracked skin behind her ears. It was sometimes uncomfortable and painful but "nothing compared to the hell Charles has been through".

Charles had severe baby acne and "sneezed a lot". He went through a rotation of standard and non-standard treatments — coconut oil, bleach baths, Vaseline, cortisone, wraps with non-stick gauze to keep the skin from being stripped — and still there were bloody sheets and misery. He reacted to yoghurt at nine months and tested positive at one year to peanuts, walnuts, egg, milk, and wheat on a combination of blood and scratch tests. He had an anaphylactic episode to walnuts at age five. After he sat in his car seat the parents would have to clean it carefully because it was covered in skin. Often, once they got in the car, he would take off his shoes and socks and scratch till he bled. Although they knew he couldn't control it, his parents constantly told him to stop scratching. Even his younger brother would tell him to stop.

At home, he would leave skin flakes and often blood stains wherever he sat or slept.

Bathing, washing, brushing — normal activities lit his skin up. They tried water filters, air filters, and only used an expensive bottled water brand, to no significant effect. It became impossible to find cleaning products, soaps, shampoos, laundry detergents, and any other body products that didn't make things worse for him. The pediatrician was very sympathetic. She said she had never seen anything like his case and sent them to specialists. The message from allergists and dermatologists was "accept that this was normal life for him". A nurse at a distinguished children's hospital told Julie that she was driving herself crazy because she was looking for answers and various ways to help him. With total IgE levels above 11,000, the allergist suggested they go to a geneticist, without any specific assurance about what that would reveal, or any therapeutic purpose. Topical steroids were applied liberally, with all the accustomed fears.

As frequently happens with patients who don't respond to conventional treatment and for whom there is no experimental treatment in prospect, the tendency is to punt them down the road. The message was always the same: "This is life for him." When his diet fell to five foods, she stopped talking to people and participating in social media groups because it seemed everyone had solutions that worked for them but not for Charles and often made things worse. It was a horror to watch her son suffer without knowing how to help him. Everyone had an opinion. In 2015, he started needing an inhaler for labored breathing. In 2015–16, and 2017, he had MRSA — a difficult-to-treat staph infection, repeatedly. He did not sleep well. They tried homeopaths and chiropractors. Her husband read about an anti-eczema diet, but a lot of the food suggestions just made matters worse.

Julie says, "I heard about Dr. Li from various groups, but was afraid of trying, yet again, something new and risking making things even worse." In the summer of 2017, Charles couldn't even wash his hands and a new blood draw showed his total IgE rising to 13,500 with most specific allergy bloodwork a class III or higher. The original Dr. Li protocol consisted of two different creams, alternating applications, every two waking hours, in addition to herbal baths, and six pills taken twice a day. While Julie's goal was to take him off topical steroids, Dr. Li counseled gradual tapering. Charles showed improvement within months. Total IgE decreased from 13,500 to

6,040 in less than five months after starting. The parents split the medication duty, with husband taking the night shift. In November 2019, Charles felt strong enough to completely stop all topical steroids.

Today Charles is "a completely different person, living a completely different life". He wears socks and shoes without complaint. He can bathe. He eats many more than five foods, hardly uses an inhaler and can sit still without itching. He sleeps sounder and can wash his hands. His body is calmer and stronger. The family is "finally confident that he is not in that horrible state and that things will not be like that forever".

30

"IT HURT TO SHOWER"

Adelina (Age 18)

Bernedeta (Adeline's mother)

Bernedeta and her husband were born in Tanzania and moved to the United States, she to study and he to work. While they lived in Long Island, their twin daughters were born.

Bernedeta says that Adelina was born with mild eczema in on her cheeks and in the folds of her legs and arms, but she didn't know what it was. She rubbed her every day with something, such as Aveeno, Desitin, or hydrocortisone. She was given oats every day, and ended up allergic to them, along with tree nuts. She itched all the time. Every early photograph shows Adelina scratching. "It hurt to shower," Adelina says, and while she loved to swim, she stopped. "By the time I was nine or ten, I couldn't bend my arms."

It should have been a wonderful childhood, with vacations in Hawaii, Dubai, and Mexico, but, Bernedeta says, "Her skin didn't look like a young girl's skin. She had white patches everywhere, swollen eyes, and sometimes purple-black blotches. Itching spread to her back and even the palms of her hands." The answer was always more hydrocortisone. A doctor called it chronic urticaria. They tried "energy healing".

Bernedeta says that Adelina developed a "dry crust" that spread to her whole body. She began shedding skin flakes, "the size of oatmeal". Wherever she sat for a time Adelina would leave a "puddle of skin", which the parents would promptly sweep up. When the family stayed in a hotel, they would decline maid service so as not to set off alarms about the health of a guest. She started sleeping all the time. She developed lesions that were dry on the outside but "like Jello inside". She stopped talking, and her twin gave her the "sleeping all day award". She lost 15 lbs. and shook all the time. When people would ask if she was cold, she would say that she was hot.

Friends who wanted to visit were warned about Adelina's appearance so they would have time to prepare. She stopped menstruating. Everything hurt, especially when she moved. She couldn't bear to look at her legs. Her skin was red and leathery. They went to a succession of alternative practitioners. An acupuncturist told her she looked like an old lady.

By this time, doctors began offering dupilumab (Dupixent), the monoclonal antibody. They went to the extent of filling out forms to initiate treatment. When Bernedeta, who had been doing her research, began to broach the idea of simultaneous treatment with Dr. Li, the doctors were dismissive. One compared it to homeopathy. "It was 'my way or the highway,'" says Bernedeta.

By the winter of 2019, Adelina was hardly going to school, although COVID-19 intervened and she was able to keep up remotely. Adelina said she was mad at the world.

Finally in September 2020, Adelina began treatment with Dr. Li. By November she could move normally. The open wounds and crust had disappeared. Her period returned. The leathery skin had given way to "new baby skin". Where she once had been reluctant to display her arms, she paraded around in tee shirts like a normal teenager. Bernedeta says of Dr. Li, "We owe our lives to her."

31

THE PARENTS WOULD LIE IN BED AND LISTEN TO HIM SCRATCH

Moshe

Chaim (Moshe's father)

Moshe's family are Hasidic Jews. When he was a few weeks old, some pimples appeared on his cheeks, which his parents thought were normal and that they would go away in time. Instead, they spread to his knees, elbows, and the rest of his face. A trip to the allergist and skin prick testing revealed sensitivity to milk and eggs, so his mother omitted them from her diet as she continued to nurse. However, the symptoms came back and continued to worsen. They began to use cortisone-based creams every three days, but as the lesions returned, they used them every other day, and then every day, but then they stopped working altogether.

A dermatologist was consulted who suggested wet pajamas and other standard measures to no avail. He woke up bloody from scratching. The parents would lie in bed and listen to him scratch. He was cranky and "never happy" for eight months. At this point, someone referred them to Dr. Xiu-Min Li, although they didn't follow through because the idea of Chinese medicine was unfamiliar. Instead, they consulted a kinesiologist for two or three months during which they used tubs of moisturizers, one of which made Moshe scream as though his skin was burning. Another kinesiologist whom they consulted in mid-2018 charged $500 a visit for a battery of tests and pronounced that it was untreatable psoriasis, but that didn't stop him from prescribing hundreds-of-dollars-worth of liquid vitamins, administered in 6–10 oral syringes daily. Every month there were new vitamins, which meant that the old ones accumulated on shelves.

The family went every summer to the Catskill Mountains where the clean air seemed to make a difference, but the fall return to Brooklyn undid the improvement. Moshe would sleep for 15 or 20 minutes at a time, but then he would resume his scratching with socks on his hands. Finally, they made an appointment with Dr. Li for six weeks but had reservations about the panels of blood work required. They spoke to their pediatrician who Googled her and was assured of her legitimacy. The blood showed sensitivity to dozens of allergens.

On their first appointment Dr. Li asked, as she always does, what they wanted to achieve. Some of it was obvious — their son was bloody. They also hoped to restore some of the staples of a Jewish diet to his life, such as nuts, certain vegetables, and baked goods. They also wanted to normalize family life. Their older child needed reassurance that Moshe commanded extra attention because he was suffering, not because he was loved more.

The initial protocol included daily 15-minute baths, ingestible tea, and two creams at two-hour intervals. The first three days showed remarkable improvement in Moshe's comfort and mood. But on day five he woke up and vomited. When he also had diarrhea, Dr. Li said no teas or bath, only the creams. During the following weeks, the diarrhea persisted and they consulted another kinesiologist who did energy testing and pronounced that Ph levels were off, prescribing lemon juice and cucumbers. They persisted with a restricted TCM protocol. Dr. Li asked that they make their own bath additives and gave them a list of herbs that were bought in Chinatown. She also gave them the name of a family in Illinois that had undergone a similar ordeal for coaching and support.

While IgE levels remained high and the gastric symptoms persisted, by the following May Moshe's skin was "almost perfect". Gastric symptoms remained and when pollen levels were high Moshe would be itchy, but overall there was tremendous progress.

32

ALL BLOOD AND CRYING

Barry

Tracy (Barry's mother)

Sydney, Australia

At the age of three weeks, Barry's skin became crusty and yellow. The doctor diagnosed an infection and prescribed an oral antibiotic and in five days the skin was clear. At eight weeks, patches of dryness and red spots began to appear, which initially were controlled with over-the-counter steroids, but subsequently covered his whole body. A pediatric dermatologist prescribed stronger steroids and moisturizers, which also worked but the symptoms returned with greater severity. Allergy tests showed sensitivity to dairy and other foods that Barry, still nursing, had never ingested, but Tracy omitted them from her diet, which didn't help.

As Barry grew, he was in "terrible pain" by mom's account. He was very weak and didn't smile. The parents covered his hands at night. He hated to go to the bathroom. Tracy confesses to having no good memories of this period of her son's life, all blood and crying.

While the parents swore off new doctors for the time being, Barry had an anaphylactic reaction and was treated at the hospital. Tracy asked an allergist assigned by the hospital if he had any thoughts about the eczema. She says, "He wouldn't go near it." Barry also had symptoms of asthma — cough or wheezing in cold weather.

Barry was so delicate that he couldn't go out. His general health was poor. As frequently happens where there is a chronically ill child, Barry absorbed so much of the mother's time that it affected the rest of the family. Her daughter complained that she spent all her time with the baby and asked her mother if she had been that attentive to her.

With the local medical environment offering no alternatives to the cyclical use of steroids and escalating outbreaks of red skin and lesions, Tracy began to search the internet and found the organization ITSAN (International Topical Steroid Addiction Network), which was formed to combat topical steroid withdrawal and red-skin syndrome. She also found a Facebook group comprised of Dr. Li's patients and their families (although not formally connected to the practice), and she read *Food Allergies: Traditional Chinese Medicine, Western Science, and the Search for a Cure*. Her family was Indonesian and familiar with the use of Chinese herbs so the extended family was open minded about it.

She discussed the possibility of going to New York for treatment with a new GP who expressed skepticism about the efficacy of the treatment and the long trip, but he agreed to order the required blood tests. Total IgE was 26,000 (<100 is normal).

Barry responded quickly to the treatment of baths, creams, and teas, although there was a difficult adjustment to the routine. Asthma improved more slowly than the skin. Recently a new tea has been added that seems to be accepted better. Ventolin is still used as needed. Nighttime wakefulness and crying improved and by six weeks his skin had cleared significantly. Total IgE has dropped to 4,000 — still high but Dr. Li points out that the actual numbers are not as important as the trend. There are no open lesions. As of the time of writing, Barry has been under treatment for 20 months. Family life has improved dramatically.

33

"WE HAVE NOTHING ELSE. GOOD LUCK"

William

Catherine (William's mother)

William was colicky. At three months, a rash appeared on the back of the child's neck and after a few weeks it became inflamed. Red spots on the face "didn't quite go away". Moisturizers and a reduced bathing schedule didn't help. The pediatrician prescribed fluticasone, and a friend who had food allergies suggested a food-elimination diet. Blood tests showed sensitivity to four out of the top eight allergens.

Dermatologists prescribed "two weeks of this, three weeks of that," according to Catherine. One doctor asked her to demonstrate her technique for applying the creams. "He wasn't sure if I was using it right." The choice of doctors was limited by her insurance. She was given the name of a pediatric dermatologist affiliated with a teaching hospital but at the appointment she never met with the dermatologist. Instead, she met with a medical student and asked if there were any alternatives to steroids, which weren't working very well. The student went away to see the unseen mentor and came back with yet another prescription for steroids. "We have nothing else. Good luck."

Catherine attempted to taper William off steroids and encountered the phenomenon of topical steroid withdrawal and red-skin syndrome. "The face was covered with red spots, the trunk was worse, and the limbs were worst of all." Cuts and scrapes were very slow to heal. It took up to three weeks to scab and so the wounds would remain open. Every night, Catherine stayed up late doing her own research. Chat groups led to a regimen of pro-biotics and a very limited diet.

Catherine comes from a Chinese family and it made sense to consult an acupuncturist, but when she did, one of the needles triggered a bad flair. The acupuncturist remarked that it made sense because treating eczema with acupuncture involved relieving the body of heat, but this had never happened before. She used an herbal tincture — one drop diluted in 10 ounces of water — but that didn't work. A holistic dermatologist suggested light therapy a few times a week, but this was incompatible with the parents' work schedules. They tried apple cider vinegar baths and mineral salts.

William had open sores and great pain. Family quality of life was "down to nothing". When William was age 20 months, a sympathetic dermatologist discussed the risks of resuming steroids vs. avoiding them altogether. Steroids would allow them to buy time. Eventually, Catherine's online research led her to Dr. Li. Although she had her doubts, conversations with patients and parents convinced her that Dr. Li was the doctor to see when nothing else worked. It was June 2016.

Upon examining William, Dr. Li said, "I have seen this before." She said, "We are going to treat this child like a burn victim." She gave Catherine a questionnaire to rate things like sleeping, eating, bowel movements, and overall quality of life on a scale of 1–10. Treatment began with a single herbal tea to be used as a bath additive. Dr. Li showed Catherine some acu-pressure points to relieve discomfort. These were things Catherine was familiar with because of her family background. Because William's digestion was very sensitive, there was to be no change in the diet for the time being. Sleep improved quickly, although night itching was the last to go. After four months, it would be okay to drink a bit of the tea at a time. At eight months they began to address the food allergies. When a cream was introduced to the regimen, it was applied to the middle of the back to keep it out of scratching range.

Three years into treatment Catherine says that there have been distinct improvements in William's health. Notably, cuts and scratches scab over right away and heal normally. Eczema flairs and hives resolve quickly. Numerous fruits and vegetables have been added to William's diet. All of the markers covered in the baseline questionnaire have improved significantly. Catherine says that William "looks like a normal kid".

34

"JUST WANTED TO BE NORMAL"

Stephen (Age 11)

Erhi (Stephen's mother)

Stephen had eczema at one year, which his mom described as "normal". His mother is a biologist and his father did a PhD at an American university. The family moved to the United States from Mongolia, and they have now lived in the US for eight years.

The eczema became a major problem when Stephen was nine. It appeared behind his knee, then spread. "He had a rash all over," says Erhi. His scalp became "one big wound" requiring hospitalization.

A pediatrician prescribed an anti-fungal treatment and a steroid shot. They worked for a couple of weeks but came back "worse and worse". During an ER visit, Stephen was given intravenous steroids.

This was taking place during the COVID-19 pandemic, so the parents were working at home. "We were miserable all the time," says Erhi. "We barely slept and took turns taking care of Stephen." Ice gel packs worked to control the itching. In the meantime, Erhi joined several Facebook groups and pursued many of the ideas she saw there, such as bleach baths, and finally came across Dr. Li's treatment. By the time they presented themselves via Zoom in December 2019, Stephen's skin was very bad, particularly his face, but they were encouraged by the confidence Dr. Li presented, which made them hopeful. Stephen "just wanted to be normal". They started on low doses of the herbal treatments while continuing oral steroids for another seven weeks. By February 2020, all signs of oozing were gone and only one spot remained behind Stephen's ear. By early March, they stopped using topical steroids.

35

"ZERO SPONTANEITY IN OUR LIVES"

James (Age 7)

Mary (James's mother)

James's mother says he had reactions to the food she ate while she breastfed him and eczema developed at about six weeks old. When he was old enough to try solid foods and get allergy testing, she realized he was a severe case. By about two years old, he had a very limited safe diet (with confirmed allergies to tree nuts, peanuts, wheat, egg, dairy, sesame, soy, garlic, and some others), debilitating eczema, and had been in the ER a few times for asthma. The parents' lives "were very much led by fear, an abundance of caution, and zero spontaneity in our lives". Despite their efforts, he had multiple food allergy reactions, and at two and a half years old he began oral immunotherapy (OIT) for tree nuts. After 6 months with ezcema flares, digestive issues, and temper changes, and no progress, they stopped OIT and began sublingual immunotherapy (SLIT) for tree nuts and peanuts.

About six months later, James had a severe anaphylactic reaction from an accidental ingestion of a small amount of baked powdered milk. At about 2 years of age, they consulted Dr. Li. Their work was initially focused on calming James's system and his severe eczema. Over 4 years, his eczema and itching cleared up, and his digestive issues were controlled.

During this period, they consulted Dr. Sanjeev Jain. Over the next three years, James was on SLIT maintenance for tree nuts and peanuts as well as

TCM with Dr. Li, and achieved OIT maintenance for wheat, dairy, egg, tree nuts, and peanuts. As he got closer to maintenance, he began to have some stomach pain, digestive issues, and more asthma flares with viruses, so Dr. Jain added to Xolair to the treatment plan. After three months of Xolair (and continued TCM and SLIT), James achieved a low-level maintenance dose for peanuts, tree nuts, dairy, and egg. Now at 7 years old James continues to have once or twice daily OIT doses, SLIT for environmentals and tree nuts, monthly Xolair, and TCM treatment. He eats wheat and baked dairy and egg freely, can eat small amounts of soy (mainly in packaged goods), and can have foods that "may contain tree nuts and peanuts".

His eczema has been gone for years and his asthma is very well controlled. Future goals are to complete environmental allergy shots and possibly build up his maintenance OIT doses to allow more free eating. Mary says, "At the moment our son is comfortable and happy with what he can eat, and his food allergies don't feel very restrictive to us."

Dr. Jain described James's case as unique and severe. It has been challenging logistically and emotionally. Mary says, "OIT treatment in particular requires caregivers to access small 'side effects' (or reactions) daily. We are now at a place where we live free, relaxed, more spontaneous lives. Our son doesn't remember the limitations his life had in his early years or much of the challenges of the OIT up-dosing time. His current treatments in maintenance are part of his daily life. At seven years old he accepts them as part of his life, much like daily tooth brushing. Our son can eat out at restaurants, sleep through the night, spend the night at friends' houses on his own, and go to birthday parties without us attending, and he can eat the cake!"

36

"A LIFE OF CHAOS AND TRAUMA"

Mark (Age 6)

Rachel (Mark's mother)

Rachel was born in Alabama, and lived in several states, but eventually she "met a Kiwi", John, and ended up settling with him in his native New Zealand where they eventually had a son, Mark.

At the age of 15 months, just before he was due for vaccinations, Mark developed bumps on his lower back, which soon spread to his whole body. The GP called it a "non-descriptive rash" and recommended that the vaccines be delayed. Hydrocortisone was given. At 18 months he was sleeping badly, and the parents had to visit him in his room to comfort him, so they brought him to sleep in their bed to hold his arms.

Treatment was managed by the GP, who eventually referred Mark to a pediatrician. In New Zealand, unlike in the United States, pediatricians are specialists rather than primary care physicians for children and there is a managed hierarchy of access. All treatment is free of charge.

By two years, his appearance had deteriorated, and strangers began commenting. Physician guidance on use of the steroids was vague, which Rachel sums up as "use when there's a rash and then stop", or "use for three days and then stop", or "use as directed". But until the age of three and a half, "frequency, intensity, and duration were increasing until we used them pretty much all the time". Mark was given betamethasone alerate under whole body wraps twice a day for five weeks. This is considered a milder corticosteroid than others, but the wrapping would amplify its potency. His skin "looked like he had been burned". Several months of methotrexate followed. This is an immune suppressant used to treat rheumatoid arthritis and psoriasis, as well as cancer of the blood, bone, lung, breast, head, and neck. The severity of Mark's condition took a terrible toll on family morale. Rachel says John was deeply depressed by watching his son suffer.

Eventually, Mark was booked to see a pediatric dermatologist from Auckland, one of only two in the country, who only visited their town twice a year. This super specialist said that steroids were dangerous in these quantities and pronounced Mark's condition as refractory. Rachel was becoming skeptical of the efficacy of the treatment. At one point, they sought some alternative therapies such as UV light, but the doctors judged he wasn't a candidate. They went to a naturopath, to no avail.

The doctors were concerned about Mark's prognosis, saying he was at risk for "severe skin infection, septicemia, cataracts due to rubbing of the eyes, Vitamin D deficiency, iron deficiency, poor growth, and the psychological effects of pain, itch, loss of sleep, and school absenteeism." Rachel had quit her job to look after Mark and began to lobby for cyclosporine, another potent immunosuppressive drug used to prevent organ rejection after transplant. However, it was not approved for refractory eczema.

Fed up with the lack of progress, after six months of methotrexate, Rachel took Mark to the Children's Hospital in Auckland and proclaimed that she wouldn't leave until he was given cyclosporine. Again, she met with resistance. At one point, staff physicians recommended a clinic in France. Eventually the drug was given. However, after two months it was agreed that it wasn't worth the risks for the benefits received.

In mid-September of 2020, Mark showed some improvement in itch and energy, although there were intense flares. To further complicate "a life of chaos and trauma", Rachel had become pregnant and had a January 2021 due date. In November of 2020, the team of doctors blamed the parents in writing for discontinuing steroid treatments and offered to see Mark again if his parents would adhere to a protocol that clearly wasn't working.

Rachel managed to connect with a woman on Facebook whose daughter had a condition like Mark's and who was also a patient of Dr. Xiu-Min Li.

Rachel was persuaded to contact Dr. Li, who gave Mark priority status for a virtual consultation as she always does with very severe cases. And upon hearing that a baby was due in January, Dr. Li insisted that treatment should begin so they could get used to the rigors of baths and creams and pills prior to the arrival of a newborn. Given the severity of Mark's condition, they expected a continuation of his sporadic day care career as kindergarten began.

Fortunately, the treatment began to work right away, for appearance, energy, and morale. He was able to handle school full time. At one Zoom meeting, Rachel told Dr. Li that Mark had a series of colds. Dr. Li lectured them sternly that not only was Mark going to school but was likely overdoing physical activity. His new life was exciting, but his immune system needed time to recover, that there was more to his health than just the condition of his skin.

At the time of writing, Rachel describes Mark as "a normal kid". It's just that part of being normal is taking lots of pills, baths, and creams. They even have found a way to explain the color of his skin from regular application of the creams. It's his "warrior paint".

Postscript

Universal free health care is a fact of life in New Zealand and TCM treatment is expensive so Mark's father initiated a petition to the Ministry of Health for reimbursement to Dr. Li going forward. The petition included the following: "To our delight, (Mark) showed quick improvement, and now having completed 3 months of treatment, his progress is excellent. When the protocol began, (Mark's) skin was affected at about 95%. Currently, his skin is mildly affected at about 10%. He is sleeping through the night for 12–13 hours every night for the first time since he was diagnosed with eczema around 17 months of age. (Mark's) scratching is akin to having a few bug bites, so dramatically different than what we have experienced over the last few years."

Their petition drew some unexpected support. Soon after Mark returned to school, he was spotted by the dermatologist whose daughter was also a student. The doctor was shocked by Mark's appearance — in a good way. He told Rachel that if he hadn't recognized Mark as the little boy with desperate eczema, he would never have guessed that there was a history of skin disease. He wrote to the Exceptional Circumstances Committee: "This is a special, complex case of a boy who has suffered for a very long time. Conventional medicines have been unsuccessful. I am not suggesting that this become the treatment for every child with eczema. This is a special case." The petition has now been accepted.

Rachel writes:

On his 4th birthday, Mark was on Methotrexate. He spent most of his party huddled in mum's lap or alone in his room scratching.

By his 5th birthday, his spirit had returned, and his condition had improved, but he was still very sick. He was no longer on immunosuppressants. He was late to his (surprise) party due to a 30-minute itch fit. He mostly enjoyed the party, with some moderate scratching and an itch fit when he arrived home. When he began school, his fine motor control was behind, as he had worn hand coverings for most of his 4th year of life. He couldn't write any letters when he started school.

Mark's obvious improvement is on the outside but the internal improvements are also documented, and outstanding. Even more, he has plumped up in his figure. Nine months ago, he was wearing size 3-4 clothing, sometimes size 5. Now, he wears 6-8. His mood is stable, he's coming off most of his conventional medications, and he's thriving. He can read and write.

Today, on his 6th birthday, he didn't itch at all. He had an "all-boys party" at a bowling alley. He ran around with his friends. He ate cake and a hot dog. He played with the neighbors when he got home. This is how his childhood should be.

INDEX

209

CPSIA information can be obtained
at www.ICGtesting.com
Printed in the USA
JSHW040304260722
28393JS00001B/54